SKIN CARE

A GUIDE TO HEALTHY AND CLEAR SKIN

BY

CHARISSA TATIANA

A GUIDE TO HEALTHY AND CLEAR SKIN

Table of Contents

INTRODUCTION

In a world where first impressions matter more than ever, the importance of healthy and clear skin cannot be overstated. "Skincare: A Guide to Healthy and Clear Skin" is a book that delves into the intricacies of skincare, offering readers a comprehensive and enlightening journey towards achieving radiant and flawless skin. In a world filled with beauty products and skincare routines, this guide is a beacon of clarity, helping readers cut through the noise and embrace a regimen that truly works.

With six decades of skincare expertise, the author, Charissa Tatiana has poured her knowledge and passion into this book. Her vast experience as a dermatologist, coupled with her dedication to demystifying skincare, makes this guide a must-read for anyone striving for that elusive healthy and clear complexion.

The book's introduction immediately sets the stage for the reader, emphasizing that skincare is not a one-size-fits-all endeavor. Each person's skin is unique, and what works for one may not work for another. Charissa Tatiana encourages readers to embrace their individuality and tailor their skincare routines accordingly. This critical insight immediately engages the reader and establishes the author as a trustworthy guide.

Charissa Tatiana navigates through the book's chapters with clarity and depth.

She delves into the fundamentals of skincare, touching on the importance of a balanced diet, proper hydration, and a good night's sleep. These are the building blocks upon which healthy and clear skin can be achieved.

One of the book's highlights is its discussion of skincare ingredients. Charissa Tatiana breaks down the myriad of components found in skincare products, offering clear explanations of what they do and how they can benefit the skin. From retinoids to hyaluronic acid, readers will gain a profound understanding of the science behind these products. This knowledge empowers individuals to make informed choices and steer clear of products that may not be suitable for their skin type.

Charissa Tatiana also addresses common skincare issues and concerns, such as acne, aging, and sun damage. Her practical advice and expert recommendations for treating these conditions are invaluable to readers seeking solutions to their skincare woes. Her emphasis on prevention as the best cure underscores the importance of establishing good habits early in one's skincare journey.

A standout feature of the book is its inclusion of personal anecdotes and case studies. Charissa Tatiana shares stories from her years in practice, revealing the transformations of patients who have followed her guidance. These real-life examples serve as inspiration and demonstrate that clear and healthy skin is within reach for anyone who is dedicated to proper skincare.

The book also provides guidance on building a personalized skincare routine. Charissa Tatiana takes the mystery out of the multi-step routines that have become so popular, offering readers a blueprint for their daily and weekly regimens. From cleansing and exfoliating to moisturizing and applying sunscreen, the steps are clearly laid out and explained, making it easy for readers to adapt these routines into their daily lives.

Additionally, "Skincare: A Guide to Healthy and Clear Skin" addresses the importance of professional skincare treatments. Charissa Tatiana discusses the benefits of dermatological procedures, like chemical peels, microdermabrasion, and laser therapy, and provides insights on when to consider these options. Her expertise in these areas assures readers that they are receiving guidance grounded in the latest advancements in skincare.

- In the final chapters, Charissa Tatiana offers invaluable advice on maintaining skin health over the long term. She reinforces the idea that skincare is a lifelong commitment and that a consistent routine, combined with the right products and treatments, can keep skin healthy and clear for years to come.

In conclusion, "Skincare: A Guide to Healthy and Clear Skin" is an indispensable resource for anyone seeking to achieve beautiful, radiant skin. Charissa Tatiana wealth of experience, dedication to clarity, and emphasis on individuality make this book a beacon of knowledge in the saturated world of skincare. With her guidance, readers can embark on a transformative journey to a healthier, happier, and more confident self. This book is not just about skincare; it's about the empowerment that comes from understanding and nurturing your own skin.

CHAPTER 1

<u>UNDERSTANDING YOUR SKIN</u>

Your skin is the largest organ in your body, serving as a protective barrier between your internal organs and the outside world. To truly care for your skin, it's essential to understand its complex nature, which goes far beyond what meets the eye.

The skin is made up of three primary layers: the epidermis, the dermis, and the subcutaneous tissue. The epidermis is the outermost layer and acts as the shield against external factors like UV radiation, pollutants, and microorganisms. Beneath the epidermis, the dermis contains vital structures such as sweat glands, hair follicles, and blood vessels. Finally, the subcutaneous tissue provides insulation and serves as a cushion against external pressure.

Your skin's appearance and health are influenced by various factors, including genetics, lifestyle, and environmental elements. By comprehending these factors, you can take better care of your skin and maintain a healthy, youthful complexion.

1. Genetics: Your genetics play a significant role in determining your skin type, including whether you have oily, dry, or combination skin. Understanding your genetic predispositions can help you choose the right skincare products and routines.

2. Skin Type: Identifying your skin type is crucial. Oily skin tends to produce excess sebum, while dry skin lacks proper moisture. Combination skin displays attributes of both oily and dry skin types. Normal skin is well-balanced. Tailoring your skincare routine to your skin type ensures you provide it with what it needs.

3. Environmental Factors: Your skin is exposed to various environmental factors daily. Excessive exposure to UV radiation from the sun may lead to premature skin aging and heighten the likelihood of developing skin cancer. Pollution can obstruct skin pores, potentially causing acne and skin irritations. Recognizing these threats allows you to take protective measures, such as applying sunscreen and cleansing your skin effectively.

4. Lifestyle Choices: Your lifestyle greatly affects your skin. Smoking, excessive alcohol consumption, and an unhealthy diet can contribute to premature aging and skin issues. Opting for a balanced diet, staying hydrated, and avoiding harmful habits can have a positive impact on your skin's appearance and health.

5. Skincare Products: Understanding the ingredients in skincare products is essential. Some ingredients, like retinol and hyaluronic acid, offer specific benefits for the skin. Others, such as fragrances and certain preservatives, can lead to irritation. Reading product labels and consulting with a dermatologist can help you make informed choices.

6. Skincare Routine: Developing a skincare routine that caters to your skin's specific needs is vital. This involves cleansing, toning, moisturizing, and protecting with sunscreen. Regularity and consistency in your routine can yield noticeable improvements in skin texture and tone.

7. Aging: As you age, your skin undergoes changes. Collagen and elastin production decreases, leading to wrinkles and sagging. Understanding the aging process can help you choose products and treatments that address these concerns.

8. Skin Conditions: Skin conditions like acne, eczema, and psoriasis require tailored care. Consult with a dermatologist to accurately diagnose and manage these conditions.

In summary, understanding your skin involves recognizing its type, genetics, the environment it faces, and your lifestyle choices. Armed with this knowledge, you can make informed decisions about skincare products, routines, and habits that will lead to healthier, more radiant skin. Your skin is your body's first line of defense, and by understanding it, you can ensure it remains a strong and resilient protector.

1.1 THE BASICS OF SKIN ANATOMY

The skin serves as an extensive protective shield, separating our internal organs from the external world, and it ranks as the body's largest organ. It is a complex and multifunctional organ, consisting of several layers and structures that work together to perform various essential functions. Understanding the basics of skin anatomy is crucial for comprehending its role in maintaining our health and well-being.

1. Epidermis: The Outermost Layer
The epidermis is the topmost layer of the skin, serving as a protective shield. It consists of multiple sub-layers, with

the outermost layer being the stratum corneum. This layer is made up of dead skin cells and acts as a barrier against external threats like UV radiation, bacteria, and chemicals.

2. Dermis: The Middle Layer
 Beneath the epidermis lies the dermis, a thicker layer that contains a network of blood vessels, hair follicles, sweat glands, and nerve endings. The dermis provides structural support to the skin and plays a crucial role in temperature regulation.

3. Subcutaneous Tissue: The Innermost Layer**
The deepest layer of the skin, often referred to as the subcutaneous tissue or hypodermis, serves as its innermost component. It consists of fat cells that

help regulate body temperature and provide cushioning and insulation.

4. Blood Vessels and Nerves

Within the dermis, a complex web of blood vessels and sensory nerves is intricately woven. Blood vessels supply nutrients and oxygen to the skin, while nerves allow us to sense various stimuli such as temperature, pressure, and pain.

5. Hair Follicles and Glands

Hair follicles are located in the dermis and are primarily responsible for the growth of hair. Attached to these follicles are sebaceous glands that produce sebum, an oily substance that helps keep the skin and hair moisturized. Additionally, there are sweat glands that release sweat, playing a vital role in thermoregulation.

6. Collagen and Elastin

The dermis also contains collagen and elastin fibers, which provide structural support to the skin. Collagen gives the skin its strength and elasticity, while elastin allows it to stretch and recoil.

7. Melanocytes and Pigmentation

Melanocytes are specialized cells in the epidermis that produce melanin, the pigment responsible for skin color. An individual's skin tone is determined by both the quantity and specific type of melanin present in their skin.

8. Immune Cells

Langerhans cells, a type of immune cell, are found in the epidermis. They help protect the skin from infections and allergies by detecting and responding to foreign substances.

9. Wound Healing

The skin has remarkable regenerative abilities. When it's injured, a series of complex processes take place to repair the damage, including inflammation, tissue rebuilding, and scar formation.

10. Skin Appendages

Skin appendages include nails, hair, and sweat glands. Nails provide protection to the fingertips and help with fine motor skills. Hair, besides its role in temperature regulation, is also a sensory organ. Sweat glands help maintain body temperature and excrete waste products.

11. Aging and Skin Changes

The skin undergoes natural aging processes, leading to changes like wrinkles, decreased elasticity, and reduced collagen production. These changes are influenced by genetic factors and environmental factors like sun exposure.

Understanding the basic anatomy of the skin is crucial for maintaining skin health and making informed choices regarding skincare and protection. Proper skincare routines, including cleansing, moisturizing, and protecting against UV radiation, can help keep the skin healthy and vibrant. Moreover, knowledge of skin anatomy is vital in the diagnosis and treatment of various skin conditions and diseases, as it provides the foundation for dermatology, the branch of medicine dedicated to skin health.

1.2 SKIN TYPES AND CHARACTERISTICS

The skin, the body's largest organ, isn't just a defensive hedge but also a reflection of one's overall health and well- being. Skin types and characteristics vary from person to person, and understanding them is pivotal for effective skincare and maintaining a healthy complexion.

There are several crucial skin types and characteristics, each with its unique features and requirements. These can astronomically be distributed into normal, dry, unctuous, combination, and sensitive skin.

Normal Skin

Normal skin is the ideal skin type that numerous people aspire to have. It's characterized by a balanced product of oil painting(sebum) and humidity, performing in skin that's neither too dry nor too unctuous. Normal skin is generally smooth, soft, and has small pores. It's lower prone to flights and mars and periods more gracefully than other skin types.

Sot Skin

Sot skin is characterized by a lack of humidity and oil painting in the skin. It frequently feels tight, rough, and may appear dull. People with dry skin may witness flakiness and greenishness, especially in cold and dry climates. It's essential to use moisturizers with hydrating constituents like hyaluronic acid to palliate blankness and maintain a healthy skin hedge.

unctuous Skin

unctuous skin is the result of hyperactive sebaceous glands, leading to inordinate oil painting product. This skin type tends to have larger pores and is prone to acne and papules due to the oil painting buildup. To manage unctuous skin, it's pivotal to use oil painting-free products and incorporate constituents like salicylic acid and niacinamide into the skincare routine to control oil painting product and help flights.

Combination Skin

Combination skin is a blend of two or further skin types on different areas of the face. For illustration, the T- zone(

forepart, nose, and chin) may be unctuous, while the cheeks are dry. Managing combination skin can be grueling since different areas bear different care. A gentle and balanced skincare routine that addresses both dry and unctuous areas is essential for maintaining healthy skin.

Sensitive Skin

Sensitive skin is prone to greenishness, vexation, and discomfort. It can be touched off by colorful factors, including harsh skincare products, environmental rudiments, or underpinning skin conditions. People with sensitive skin should conclude for scent-free, hypoallergenic products and patch- test new products before applying them to their entire face.

In addition to these primary skin types, there are colorful skin characteristics that impact its appearance and condition.

Aging Skin

As we progress, the skin undergoes colorful changes, similar as dropped collagen product, which leads to wrinkles and sagging. The key to managing growing skin is using products withanti-aging constituents like retinol and antioxidants and guarding the skin from sun damage with sunscreen.

Acne- Prone Skin

Acne-prone skin is susceptible to frequent flights and mars. Effective skincare routines for this skin type should include products containing salicylic acid, benzoyl peroxide, or glycolic acid to control acne.

Hyperpigmented Skin

Hyperpigmentation refers to dark spots or patches on the skin, frequently caused by sun exposure or hormonal changes. To manage hyperpigmented skin, products with constituents like vitamin C and niacinamide can help fade dark spots and indeed out skin tone.

Understanding your skin type and characteristics is the first step in maintaining healthy and radiant skin. While genetics play a significant part in determining your skin type, environmental factors and proper skincare routines can greatly impact how your skin looks and feels.

Customizing your skincare routine to meet your specific skin type and addressing individual characteristics is the key to achieving and maintaining beautiful, healthy skin throughout your life.

CHAPTER 2

THE IMPORTANCE OF SKIN CARE

Skin care is a topic of increasing significance in our lives, as it plays a vital role in maintaining our overall health and well-being. Our skin serves as the body's first line of defense against external elements, making it imperative to understand and acknowledge the importance of proper skin care.

First and foremost, skin care is essential for maintaining the health and integrity of our skin. The skin is the body's largest organ and acts as a barrier, protecting us from harmful microorganisms, UV radiation, and environmental pollutants. Without proper care, the skin can become dry, damaged, and prone to various skin conditions, such as acne, eczema, and dermatitis. Neglecting skin care can lead to these conditions, causing discomfort and sometimes even long-term health issues.

Additionally, skin care is closely linked to self-esteem and confidence. Clear, healthy skin enhances one's physical appearance and can significantly boost self-esteem. When individuals feel good about their skin, they are more likely to feel confident and positive about themselves. Conversely, skin problems can lead to a decrease in self-confidence and social anxiety. Therefore, maintaining proper skin care routines can have a direct impact on one's mental well-being.

Furthermore, good skin care practices can help in delaying the signs of aging. Wrinkles, fine lines, and age spots are common skin issues associated with the aging process. By following a consistent skin care routine, individuals can slow down the appearance of these signs, giving them a more youthful and vibrant complexion. Using sunscreen, moisturizers, and anti-aging products can be particularly effective in this regard.

Skin care also plays a significant role in preventing skin cancer. Prolonged exposure to UV rays from the sun or tanning beds can increase the risk of skin cancer. Proper skin care includes the regular use of sunscreen, protective clothing, and the avoidance of excessive sun exposure, all of which are crucial in reducing this risk.

Beyond health and appearance, skin care contributes to one's overall comfort. Proper hydration and moisturization can alleviate dry and itchy skin, while the use of gentle cleansers can prevent irritation. Skin conditions like eczema and psoriasis can be managed more effectively with the right skin care regimen, minimizing discomfort and itchiness.

In conclusion, skin care is of paramount importance, as it encompasses aspects of health, self-esteem, confidence, and overall well-being. By taking steps to protect and nourish our skin, we can not only prevent various skin conditions but also enhance our physical appearance, boost self-confidence, and support our mental health. Proper skin care is a proactive approach to maintaining our health and quality of life, and it should be regarded as an essential part of our daily routine.

2.1 WHY SKIN CARE MATTERS

Skin care is a topic that has gained increasing importance in recent years, and for good reason. Beyond the realm of vanity, skin care is a fundamental aspect of our overall health and well-being. It matters for a multitude of reasons, both aesthetic and functional, and its significance cannot be overstated.

First and foremost, skin care plays a pivotal role in maintaining healthy skin. The skin, as the body's largest organ, plays a crucial role in shielding us from the external environment. It provides protection against damaging UV rays, pollutants, and pathogens. Neglecting proper skin care can lead to various skin issues, such as acne, dryness, and premature aging. By adhering to a regular skin care routine, you can cleanse, moisturize, and protect your skin, thereby preventing or mitigating these problems.

Furthermore, skin care is vital for promoting a youthful appearance. The aging process is inevitable, but with the right skin care practices, you can slow down the signs of aging. Products like sunscreen, antioxidants, and retinoids can help reduce the appearance of wrinkles, fine lines, and age spots. A well-maintained skin care regimen can boost your self-esteem and confidence, allowing you to feel comfortable in your own skin.

Beyond aesthetics, skin care also contributes to overall health. Skin conditions can be more than just a cosmetic concern. Eczema, psoriasis, and dermatitis are just a few examples of skin disorders that can cause discomfort and even pain. Proper skin care can alleviate symptoms and improve the quality of life for those affected by these conditions.

Skin care also serves as a form of self-care. Taking the time to cleanse, moisturize, and pamper your skin can be a therapeutic and soothing ritual. It provides a moment of respite in our busy lives and allows for self-reflection and relaxation. Engaging in a skin care routine can be a form of mindfulness, helping to reduce stress and promote mental well-being.

In addition, the importance of skin care extends to maintaining a balanced skin microbiome. The skin is home to a diverse community of microorganisms that play a vital role in protecting against harmful bacteria and maintaining healthy skin. Overusing harsh products or neglecting skin care can disrupt this delicate balance, leading to skin issues. By using appropriate products and techniques, you can support a harmonious skin microbiome.

In a world where beauty standards have been heavily influenced by social media and advertising, skin care serves as a reminder that beauty is not solely defined by appearance but also by the care we invest in ourselves. This shift in perspective has led to a growing trend of self-acceptance and embracing natural beauty. Skin care empowers individuals to take control of their own narrative and redefine beauty on their terms.

In conclusion, skin care matters for a multitude of reasons. It is essential for maintaining healthy skin, promoting a youthful appearance, and preventing skin conditions. Beyond the physical benefits, it is a form of self-care that contributes to mental well-being. By adopting a conscientious skin care routine, you not only take care of your skin but also take a step towards holistic well-being. Skin care is not just about looking good; it's about feeling good in your own skin and embracing your unique beauty.

2.2 COMMON SKIN ISSUES

When skin issues arise, they can be not only physically uncomfortable but also emotionally distressing. Psoriasis is one such common skin issue that affects millions of people worldwide. We will delve into the intricacies of psoriasis, shedding light on its causes, symptoms, and available treatments.

UNDERSTANDING PSORIASIS

Psoriasis is a chronic inflammatory skin disorder characterized by an accelerated production of skin cells, resulting in a buildup of cells on the skin's surface. These excess skin cells form scales and red patches that are sometimes itchy and painful. While the exact cause of psoriasis remains a subject of ongoing research, it is widely believed to be a result of genetic and environmental factors. If you have a family history of psoriasis, you might be more susceptible to developing the condition.

COMMON SYMPTOMS OF PSORIASIS

Psoriasis is known for its diverse range of symptoms, but the most common manifestations include:

1. **Red Patches:** These patches are often covered with silvery scales and can appear on any part of the body, though they frequently affect the elbows, knees, and scalp.

2. Itching and Burning: Psoriasis can be intensely itchy and, in some cases, cause a burning sensation, making it difficult to resist scratching.

3. Thickened or Pitted Nails: Psoriasis can also affect the nails, causing them to become thickened, discolored, or develop small pits.

4. Joint Pain: In some individuals, psoriasis can lead to a type of arthritis known as psoriatic arthritis, which results in joint pain and swelling.

5. Dry Cracked Skin: The condition often leads to dry, cracked skin that may bleed or become painful.

6. Inverse Psoriasis: This type of psoriasis appears as red and inflamed lesions in skin folds, such as the armpits, under the breasts, or in the genital area.

TREATMENT OPTIONS

While psoriasis is a chronic condition with no known cure, various treatment options are available to manage its symptoms and improve the quality of life for those affected:

1. **Topical Treatments:** These include creams, ointments, and shampoos containing corticosteroids, retinoids, or coal tar. They can help reduce inflammation, itching, and the buildup of skin cells.

2. **Phototherapy:** Ultraviolet (UV) light can slow down the growth of skin cells.

In phototherapy, the skin is exposed to controlled amounts of UVB or UVA light to manage psoriasis symptoms.

3. Oral Medications: In more severe cases, doctors may prescribe oral medications like methotrexate, cyclosporine, or newer biologics. These medications work to suppress the immune system's overreaction, which is a key factor in psoriasis.

4. Lifestyle and Dietary Adjustments: Some individuals find relief from psoriasis symptoms through lifestyle changes, such as maintaining a healthy weight, reducing stress, and avoiding triggers like smoking and excessive alcohol consumption.

5. Moisturizers: Regular application of moisturizers can help soothe and hydrate the skin, reducing the risk of dryness, cracking, and discomfort.

6. Biologics: These newer medications, often prescribed for moderate to severe psoriasis, target specific parts of the immune system to reduce inflammation.

EMOTIONAL IMPACT

Psoriasis is not just a physical condition; it can have a significant emotional impact. Living with visible skin lesions can lead to feelings of self-consciousness and a diminished quality of life. Those affected may experience depression, anxiety, and a reduced sense of self-esteem. It's essential to recognize and address the emotional aspects of psoriasis and seek support when needed.

In conclusion, psoriasis is a complex skin issue that affects millions of people worldwide. Understanding its causes, symptoms, and treatment options is crucial for both individuals dealing with psoriasis and the general public. While there is no cure, various treatments can help manage the symptoms and improve the overall quality of life for those affected. Moreover, addressing the emotional impact and seeking support is a vital aspect of managing this chronic condition. Psoriasis, with its visible and often uncomfortable symptoms, highlights the importance of empathy, understanding, and medical research in the realm of common skin issues.

CHAPTER 3

BUILDING YOUR SKIN CARE ROUTINE

However, it is susceptible to a wide range of diseases, conditions, and issues that can affect its appearance and health. Building a skin care routine tailored to specific skin diseases is essential in managing and improving these conditions. In this 600-word guide, we will explore the key principles of creating a personalized skin care routine for common skin diseases.

Before delving into skin care routines, it's crucial to have a basic understanding of the common skin diseases and conditions you might be dealing with.

These can include acne, eczema, psoriasis, rosacea, and more. Each condition has its own unique symptoms, triggers, and management requirements, making personalized care a necessity.

CONSULT A DERMATOLOGIST

The first step in building a skin care routine for skin diseases is to consult a dermatologist. A dermatologist can provide a precise diagnosis of your skin condition and recommend suitable treatments and products. They can also help identify any underlying causes or triggers for your skin condition.

CLEANSING

Proper cleansing is the foundation of any skin care routine, regardless of the specific skin disease. Use a gentle, soap-free cleanser that matches your skin type. For sensitive skin prone to conditions like eczema, choose a cleanser with minimal fragrance and additives. For acne-prone skin, consider a cleanser containing salicylic acid or benzoyl peroxide.

MOISTURIZERS

Skin diseases often lead to dry, flaky, or inflamed skin. Moisturizing is essential to help maintain the skin's natural barrier. Look for a fragrance-free, hypoallergenic moisturizer. For eczema or psoriasis, moisturizers containing ceramides can be particularly helpful in repairing the skin barrier.

MEDICATED TREATMENTS

Depending on your skin disease, you may need to incorporate medicated treatments. These can include topical creams, ointments, or oral medications prescribed by your dermatologist. For example, retinoids are often used for acne, while corticosteroids may be prescribed for eczema. It's essential to follow your dermatologist's instructions for the proper application and usage of these medications.

SUN PROTECTION

Sun protection is a vital component of any skin care routine. Skin diseases can make the skin more susceptible to UV damage. Make sure to use a broad-spectrum sunscreen with a minimum SPF of 30 every day, regardless of cloud cover. For those with extremely sensitive skin, consider physical sunscreens containing zinc oxide or titanium dioxide.

AVOID TRIGGERS

Recognize and steer clear of factors that exacerbate your skin condition. For example, if you have rosacea, alcohol, spicy foods, and extreme temperatures can exacerbate symptoms. If you have contact dermatitis, identify and avoid products or substances that cause irritation.

SPECIALIZED PRODUCTS

Certain skin diseases may benefit from specialized products. For instance, those with rosacea may find relief in products with anti-inflammatory ingredients like niacinamide or azelaic acid. People with psoriasis might opt for products with salicylic acid to manage scaling and flaking.

HYDRATION AND DIET

Good skin health begins from the inside out. Maintaining proper hydration and adhering to a well-balanced diet that's abundant in antioxidants, vitamins, and essential minerals is vital for overall health. Certain foods, like fatty fish with omega-3 fatty acids, can help reduce inflammation associated with skin diseases.

REGULAR FOLLOW-UPS

Skin conditions can change over time, so it's essential to have regular follow-up appointments with your dermatologist. They can adjust your skin care routine and treatment plan as needed.

PATIENCE AND CONSISTENCY

Managing skin diseases is often a long-term process. Be consistent and patient with your skin care routine. It may take time to see improvements, but maintaining a regular regimen is key to achieving healthier skin.

In conclusion, building a skin care routine for skin diseases is a personalized journey that requires careful consideration, professional guidance, and patience. Understanding your skin condition, consulting a dermatologist, and selecting the right products are crucial steps in managing and improving the health of your skin. By following a tailored routine and making lifestyle adjustments, you can achieve healthier, more radiant skin, even in the presence of skin diseases.

3.1 CREATING A DAILY ROUTINE

Creating a daily routine is a powerful way to structure your day, enhance productivity, and achieve your goals. Whether you're a student, a professional, or someone seeking a healthier lifestyle, a well-thought-out daily routine can make a significant difference in your life.

The first step in creating a daily routine is to identify your goals and priorities. What do you want to accomplish? This could range from completing work tasks to finding time for hobbies and self-care. Once you have a clear understanding of your objectives, you can tailor your routine to align with them.

Time management is a crucial aspect of any daily routine. It's important to allocate time for essential tasks, such as work or studying, and also for relaxation and self-care. Begin by setting fixed times for waking up and going to bed. A consistent sleep schedule can improve your overall health and energy levels.

To maximize your productivity, organize your day by breaking it into time blocks. For instance, allocate focused work time in the morning when you're most alert and creative. Use this time to tackle complex tasks and projects. In the afternoon, schedule less demanding tasks or meetings. Finally, set aside time in the evening for winding down and preparing for the next day.

Don't forget to incorporate breaks into your routine. Short breaks can refresh your mind and help prevent burnout. You may also explore the concept of time blocking, where you allocate specific chunks of time to focused work and then build in short, rejuvenating breaks between those intervals.

Prioritize self-care and physical activity. Include time for exercise, meditation, or relaxation techniques in your routine. Taking care of your physical and mental health is vital for maintaining your overall well-being.

Nutrition is another essential aspect of daily life. Plan your meals and snacks, ensuring they provide the necessary nutrients to sustain your energy levels.

Avoid skipping meals or relying too heavily on processed foods.

A well-structured daily routine should also include time for learning and personal growth. Whether it's reading, taking courses, or practicing a new skill, continuous learning can be transformative. Allocate time for these activities regularly.

Flexibility is key. Life is full of uncertainties, and unforeseen circumstances can easily throw off your carefully planned schedule. Stay open to making schedule changes as the situation demands. Instead of getting discouraged, view such disruptions as opportunities for adaptability and resilience.

Maintain a clean and organized workspace. A clutter-free environment can boost your efficiency and focus. Make it a part of your daily routine to tidy up your workspace before and after work or study sessions.

Lastly, self-assessment is essential for refining your daily routine. Regularly evaluate your productivity and well-being. Are you achieving your goals? Are there areas where your routine could be more efficient or fulfilling? Adjust your routine as needed to continually improve it.

In conclusion, creating a daily routine is a dynamic process that requires thoughtful planning, consistency, and flexibility. A well-designed routine can help you achieve your goals, enhance your productivity, and improve your overall quality of life. By incorporating time management, self-care, nutrition, and learning, you can develop a routine that maximizes your potential while maintaining your physical and mental well-being. Regular self-assessment ensures that your routine remains aligned with your objectives, allowing you to adapt and thrive in an ever-changing world.

3.2 SPECIALIZED TREATMENTS FOR YOUR SKIN

Skin diseases can significantly impact one's quality of life, causing discomfort, embarrassment, and sometimes even pain. Fortunately, specialized treatments tailored to specific skin conditions have evolved over the years, providing effective relief and restoration. These treatments target a wide range of skin diseases, from common issues like acne and eczema to more severe conditions such as psoriasis and vitiligo.

Acne is a prevalent skin condition, affecting people of all ages. Specialized treatments often include topical creams or gels with ingredients like benzoyl peroxide or salicylic acid to reduce inflammation and prevent breakouts. For severe cases, dermatologists may recommend oral antibiotics, hormonal therapy, or even isotretinoin. Laser therapy and chemical peels are other options for acne scarring.

Eczema, or atopic dermatitis, is characterized by itchy, red, and inflamed skin. Specialized treatments aim to alleviate these symptoms and prevent flare-ups. Moisturizers, topical corticosteroids, and calcineurin inhibitors are commonly prescribed. In severe cases, phototherapy or biologics may be recommended.

Psoriasis is a chronic skin condition that results in thick, red, and scaly patches. Specialized treatments include topical corticosteroids, phototherapy, and systemic medications. Biologics, which target specific parts of the immune system, have revolutionized psoriasis treatment, offering remarkable results for many patients.

Vitiligo is a condition in which the skin loses its pigmentation, resulting in white patches. Specialized treatments can help to repigment the skin. Topical corticosteroids, calcineurin inhibitors, and narrowband ultraviolet B (NB-UVB) phototherapy are commonly used. Surgical options like skin grafting or microskin grafting can be considered in some cases.

Rosacea manifests as persistent facial redness accompanied by prominent blood vessels on the skin's surface. Specialized treatments may include topical or oral antibiotics, as well as topical creams to reduce redness. Laser therapy is also effective in managing symptoms.

Skin cancer, while not a disease in the traditional sense, is a life-threatening condition that requires specialized treatments. Depending on the type and stage of skin cancer, treatments may involve surgical removal, radiation therapy, or immunotherapy.

Melasma causes brown or gray-brown patches on the skin, often as a result of sun exposure or hormonal changes. Specialized treatments include topical depigmenting agents, chemical peels, and laser therapy.

Hives, or urticaria, lead to itchy welts on the skin. Specialized treatments may involve antihistamines, corticosteroids, or epinephrine for severe cases. Identifying and avoiding triggers is essential for long-term management.

Specialized treatments for skin diseases should always be tailored to the individual, taking into account factors such as the type and severity of the condition, skin type, and medical history. Dermatologists are trained to assess these factors and develop a personalized treatment plan.

In addition to medical treatments, maintaining a healthy skincare routine and practicing sun protection can help prevent and manage many skin conditions. Consulting a dermatologist is crucial to ensure the best outcomes, as they can provide expert guidance on specialized treatments and ongoing care for various skin diseases. Remember, your skin is unique, and so should be your approach to its care and treatment.

CHAPTER 4

CLEANSING YOUR SKIN

Cleansing your skin is a fundamental step in any skincare routine, and its importance cannot be overstated. Our skin is our body's largest organ, and it serves as the first line of defense against environmental toxins, pathogens, and the harsh effects of daily living. As such, maintaining clean and healthy skin is not only essential for our overall well-being but also for achieving a radiant and youthful complexion.

One of the primary reasons why cleansing is crucial is to remove impurities that accumulate on the skin's surface throughout the day. These impurities can include dirt, dust, makeup, sweat, and excess oil. If left on the skin, they can clog pores and lead to various skin issues, such as acne, blackheads, and dullness. Therefore, cleansing your skin helps to unclog pores, preventing breakouts and promoting a clearer complexion.

Furthermore, effective cleansing plays a significant role in maintaining the skin's natural moisture balance. The skin has a delicate barrier called the acid mantle, which consists of natural oils and beneficial bacteria. This barrier protects the skin from external aggressors while preventing excessive moisture loss. Harsh cleansers or neglecting to cleanse can disrupt this balance, leading to dryness, sensitivity, and irritation. Using a gentle, pH-balanced cleanser helps maintain this vital barrier, ensuring the skin remains healthy and hydrated.

Selecting the appropriate cleanser tailored to your unique skin type is of utmost importance. For those with oily or acne-prone skin, a foaming or gel cleanser that contains salicylic acid or benzoyl peroxide can be effective in controlling excess oil and preventing breakouts. On the other hand, people with dry or sensitive skin should opt for a hydrating or cream cleanser that doesn't strip the skin of its natural oils.

Besides daily cleansing, it's also crucial to consider the importance of nighttime cleansing. Throughout the day, your skin comes into contact with environmental pollutants, UV rays, and other irritants. Nighttime cleansing not only removes these impurities but also helps prepare the skin for the rejuvenating process that occurs during sleep. This is when skin cells repair and regenerate, and a clean canvas ensures better results from your skincare products.

In addition to its physical benefits, the act of cleansing can be a relaxing and meditative part of your daily routine. Taking a few minutes in the morning and evening to care for your skin can be a form of self-care, reducing stress and promoting overall well-being. Using a warm washcloth or a cleansing brush can make the process even more enjoyable and effective.

In conclusion, cleansing your skin is a fundamental step in skincare that should not be underestimated. It goes beyond the simple act of removing dirt and makeup; it's about maintaining the health and beauty of your skin. By choosing the right cleanser for your skin type, being consistent with your routine, and understanding the importance of nighttime cleansing, you can achieve a clear, radiant complexion that reflects your overall well-being. Make cleansing a priority in your skincare regimen, and your skin will thank you with a healthy, glowing appearance.

4.1 CLEANSERS AND THEIR TYPES

Toners play a crucial role in maintaining a healthy skincare regimen. They play a crucial role in removing dirt, oil, makeup, and impurities from the skin's surface, helping to maintain a healthy complexion. With a wide variety of cleansers available, it's important to understand the different types and their unique benefits.

1. Gel Cleansers: Gel cleansers are water-based and often contain ingredients like glycerin. They are excellent for individuals with oily or combination skin, as they effectively remove excess sebum without over-drying the skin. Gel cleansers provide a refreshing and clean feeling, making them popular in warm weather.

2. Foaming Cleansers: These cleansers start as a gel or cream and transform into a foamy lather when mixed with water. They are excellent for removing makeup and impurities, leaving the skin feeling clean and refreshed. However, they can be a bit harsh and drying for those with dry or sensitive skin.

3. Cream Cleansers: Cream cleansers are gentle and moisturizing. They are ideal for individuals with dry or sensitive skin, as they don't strip the skin of its natural oils. These cleansers often contain ingredients like aloe vera and chamomile to soothe the skin.

4. Oil Cleansers: Oil cleansers are perfect for removing stubborn makeup and sunscreen. They work on the principle that "like dissolves like." By using an oil-based cleanser, you can effectively dissolve the oils in your makeup and cleanse your skin without stripping it of its natural moisture. Oil cleansers can be a great choice for all skin types.

5. Micellar Water: Micellar water is a gentle, water-based cleanser that contains tiny oil molecules (micelles) suspended in water. These micelles attract and remove impurities, making it an excellent option for quick and gentle cleansing, especially for those with sensitive skin.

6. Balm Cleansers: Balm cleansers are rich and luxurious. They are perfect for those who wear heavy makeup or waterproof sunscreen. These cleansers melt into an oil-like consistency upon contact with the skin, effectively dissolving makeup and impurities. They are often followed by a second, water-based cleanser to ensure a thorough clean.

7. Clay Cleansers: Clay cleansers contain various types of clay, such as kaolin or bentonite. They are excellent for deep cleansing and purifying the skin. Clay cleansers can help absorb excess oil, unclog pores, and exfoliate the skin gently.

8. Exfoliating Cleansers: Exfoliating cleansers contain small particles or acids like alpha hydroxy acids (AHAs) or beta hydroxy acids (BHAs) to slough away dead skin cells. They help improve skin texture and promote cell turnover. However, they should be used with caution, as overuse can lead to skin sensitivity.

9. Powder Cleansers: Powder cleansers are dry, powdered formulations that are activated with water. They are versatile and customizable, allowing you to adjust the level of exfoliation based on the amount of water used. Powder cleansers often contain enzymes or mild exfoliants.

Choosing the right cleanser is crucial for your skin's health and appearance. It's essential to consider your skin type, concerns, and any specific issues when selecting a cleanser. Experimenting with different types can help you find the perfect match for your skincare routine. Additionally, it's important to follow your cleanser with a suitable moisturizer to maintain your skin's hydration and balance. Proper cleansing is the foundation of healthy, radiant skin.

4.2 THE ART OF PROPER CLEANSING

Cleansing is an essential step in any skincare routine, serving as the foundation upon which healthy and radiant skin is built. Proper cleansing not only helps maintain clear and beautiful skin but also plays a crucial role in preventing and managing various skin diseases.

Cleansing, at its core, involves the removal of dirt, excess oil, makeup, and environmental pollutants from the skin's surface. This seemingly simple step holds profound importance in both daily skincare and the management of skin diseases.

DAILY CLEANSING AND SKIN HEALTH

Every day, our skin faces a barrage of challenges, from air pollution to sweat and oil production. These impurities can accumulate on the skin's surface, leading to clogged pores, acne, and an uneven complexion. By cleansing the skin, you effectively eliminate these unwanted elements, allowing your skin to breathe and function optimally.

The art of daily cleansing starts with choosing the right cleanser for your skin type. For those with oily skin, a gentle foaming cleanser can help control excess sebum production. On the other hand, individuals with dry or sensitive skin may benefit from a hydrating, cream-based cleanser that retains moisture. It's crucial to strike a balance; overly harsh cleansers can strip the skin of its natural oils, leading to irritation and dryness.

Incorporating the correct cleansing technique is equally important. Gently massage the cleanser onto your skin using circular motions and rinse with lukewarm water. Steer clear of scalding hot water, as it can be abrasive to your skin. After cleansing, pat your skin dry with a clean towel instead of rubbing, which can cause unnecessary friction and irritation.

CLEANSING AND SKIN DISEASE MANAGEMENT

Cleansing plays an integral role in managing various skin diseases. For those with acne-prone skin, it helps to remove excess oil and impurities that can clog pores and contribute to breakouts. A consistent cleansing routine is often a fundamental part of dermatologists' recommendations for acne management.

Skin diseases like eczema and psoriasis benefit from the gentle cleansing of the affected areas. Using a mild, fragrance-free cleanser can prevent further irritation and help maintain the skin's moisture balance. Proper cleansing is a preparatory step that allows medications and treatments to be more effectively absorbed, offering relief to those suffering from chronic skin conditions.

Skin diseases like fungal infections often require special care, including antifungal cleansers. Proper cleansing is essential in removing fungal spores from the skin's surface and reducing the risk of recurrence.

Moreover, individuals with skin diseases need to be particularly mindful of their cleansing habits. Harsh or irritating cleansers can exacerbate symptoms. Therefore, it's crucial to consult with a dermatologist to determine the most suitable products and routines tailored to specific skin conditions.

In conclusion, the art of proper cleansing is a fundamental aspect of both daily skincare and the management of skin diseases. By selecting the right cleanser, employing a gentle technique, and adapting the routine to your unique skin type and condition, you can maintain healthy, radiant skin, prevent problems, and aid in the management of various skin diseases. It's a small but powerful step that forms the basis for your skin's overall health and beauty.

CHAPTER 5

MOISTURIZERS AND HYDRATION

Proper skincare goes beyond cleansing and treating skin conditions. Hydration, often in the form of moisturizers, is a vital component in the battle against various skin diseases. Whether you're dealing with dryness, eczema, psoriasis, or other dermatological issues, understanding the significance of moisturization can make a substantial difference in your skin's health and overall well-being.

THE ROLE OF MOISTURIZERS IN SKIN HEALTH

Moisturizers are not just cosmetic products; they are essential for maintaining the skin's natural protective barrier. This protective barrier consists of lipids and water, and when it's compromised, the skin becomes more susceptible to irritation, infections, and the development of skin diseases. Moisturizers serve as a crucial tool in restoring and preserving this barrier.

For individuals with dry skin, using a moisturizer helps replenish lost moisture and reinforces the skin's barrier function. Dry skin can be more prone to itching, flaking, and developing eczema or dermatitis, making moisturization a critical part of prevention.

ECZEMA AND PSORIASIS: THE HYDRATION CONNECTION

Eczema and psoriasis are chronic skin diseases that can be challenging to manage. Both conditions are characterized by symptoms such as itching, inflammation, and dry, scaly skin. Proper hydration is key in alleviating these symptoms and reducing the frequency and severity of flare-ups.

In the case of eczema, which often affects children and adults, a moisturizer should be applied immediately after bathing. This locks in moisture and helps repair the skin barrier, reducing the itch-scratch cycle. Moreover, choosing a moisturizer that is fragrance-free and hypoallergenic is essential for preventing further irritation.

Psoriasis, another autoimmune skin condition, benefits from well-hydrated skin. While moisturizers alone may not treat psoriasis, they can help alleviate the discomfort and scaling associated with the condition. Combined with appropriate medical treatments, moisturization plays a supporting role in managing the disease.

SELECTING THE RIGHT MOISTURIZER

Choosing the right moisturizer is crucial when dealing with skin diseases. For sensitive skin or skin prone to dermatological issues, opt for products with minimal ingredients, avoiding fragrances and harsh chemicals. Look for moisturizers that contain ceramides, hyaluronic acid, or glycerin, as these ingredients aid in repairing the skin's barrier and retaining moisture.

In extremely dry or eczema-prone skin, ointments are often recommended. They provide a thicker, more effective barrier, sealing in moisture and providing relief from dryness and itching.

HYDRATION FROM WITHIN

While topical moisturization is vital, internal hydration is just as essential. Drinking an adequate amount of water is essential for overall skin health. Proper hydration from within helps maintain skin elasticity and assists in flushing out toxins that can exacerbate skin diseases.

In conclusion, moisturizers and proper hydration are indispensable tools in the management and prevention of skin diseases. They assist in restoring and maintaining the skin's protective barrier, reducing symptoms like dryness, itching, and inflammation. When dealing with conditions like eczema and psoriasis, combining appropriate medical treatments with the right moisturization routine can significantly improve the quality of life for those affected by these skin diseases. The path to healthier skin often begins with a well-chosen moisturizer and a commitment to maintaining proper hydration.

5.1 BENEFITS OF HYDRATION

Proper hydration is a fundamental aspect of maintaining overall health, and its impact on skin health, particularly in the context of skin diseases, cannot be overstated. The skin, the body's largest organ, serves as a vital barrier against external threats and plays a crucial role in temperature regulation, immune response, and detoxification. When the body lacks sufficient hydration, the skin is one of the first organs to suffer, and this can exacerbate or even lead to various skin diseases. Here, we delve into the numerous benefits of hydration in relation to skin diseases.

1. Improved Skin Barrier Function: Hydration is essential for maintaining the skin's barrier function. A well-hydrated skin barrier is more resilient and better equipped to defend against environmental pollutants and pathogens. Dehydrated skin is prone to becoming compromised, allowing irritants to penetrate, potentially leading to conditions like eczema or contact dermatitis.

2. Enhanced Wound Healing: Skin diseases, injuries, or surgical procedures often leave the skin in need of repair. Proper hydration facilitates efficient wound healing by increasing blood flow and nutrient delivery to the affected area, reducing the risk of complications like infection and scarring.

3. Minimized Itchiness and Inflammation: Skin diseases, such as psoriasis or dry skin, often manifest with symptoms like itchiness and inflammation. Hydration can alleviate these discomforts by preventing excessive dryness and reducing the irritation associated with these conditions.

4. Regulation of Oil Production: Acne and other oil-related skin disorders can be exacerbated by dehydrated skin. Paradoxically, dry skin can trigger the sebaceous glands to produce more oil, which can clog pores and lead to breakouts. Adequate hydration helps to regulate oil production and prevent acne flare-ups.

5. Maintenance of Skin Elasticity: Hydration contributes to skin's suppleness and elasticity. As we age, the skin naturally loses its elasticity, leading to wrinkles and sagging. Proper hydration can slow down this process, making the skin more resilient against the development of fine lines and wrinkles.

6. Detoxification and Clearer Complexion: A well-hydrated body is more efficient at flushing out toxins, which can otherwise accumulate in the skin and lead to conditions like rashes or acne. Hydration assists in maintaining a clearer, healthier complexion.

7. Protection Against UV Damage: Chronic dehydration can render the skin more susceptible to damage from UV radiation. Adequately hydrated skin is better equipped to handle sun exposure, reducing the risk of sunburn and skin diseases like skin cancer.

8. Improvement in Skin Conditions: In many cases, skin diseases are exacerbated by dehydration. Conditions like dermatitis, rosacea, and psoriasis often become less severe or easier to manage when the skin is well-hydrated.

9. Boosted Collagen Production: Collagen is a key structural protein that keeps the skin youthful and firm. Hydration is essential for the production of collagen, which can help mitigate the signs of aging and keep the skin healthier overall.

In conclusion, maintaining proper hydration is a simple yet powerful means of promoting skin health and preventing or alleviating skin diseases. Dehydrated skin is more susceptible to damage, inflammation, and disease, while well-hydrated skin is resilient and better equipped to defend against external threats. Ensuring adequate water intake, using moisturizers, and adopting a skin-friendly diet can go a long way in preventing and managing various skin conditions. In this context, hydration is not just a matter of cosmetic concern but a fundamental component of overall health and well-being.

5.2 SUN PROTECTION AND SKIN HEALTH

Sun protection is an essential component of maintaining healthy skin and plays a critical role in preventing various skin diseases. Exposure to the sun's harmful ultraviolet (UV) rays can lead to a range of skin conditions, including skin cancer, premature aging, and exacerbation of existing skin diseases. Understanding the importance of sun protection is key to safeguarding skin health.

1. Skin Cancer Prevention: Perhaps the most significant benefit of sun protection is the prevention of skin cancer. Prolonged and unprotected sun exposure is a leading cause of skin

cancer, including melanoma, squamous cell carcinoma, and basal cell carcinoma. Regular use of sunscreen and protective clothing can significantly reduce the risk of developing these life-threatening conditions.

2. Preventing Premature Aging: UV rays from the sun accelerate the aging of the skin. This includes the formation of wrinkles, fine lines, age spots, and loss of skin elasticity. By shielding your skin from the sun, you can maintain a more youthful appearance and delay the onset of these aging signs.

3. Minimized Risk of Sunburn: Sunburns are not only painful but also damaging to the skin. Severe sunburns can cause blisters, peeling, and an increased risk of skin diseases like skin cancer.

Sunscreen and avoiding the sun during peak hours can prevent sunburns and their associated complications.

4. Reduction in Hyperpigmentation: Prolonged sun exposure can lead to hyperpigmentation, causing dark patches or uneven skin tone. Conditions like melasma can worsen with sun exposure. Sun protection, including sunscreen and protective clothing, can help prevent or reduce hyperpigmentation.

5. Protection for Sensitive Skin: Individuals with sensitive skin or certain skin diseases, such as rosacea or eczema, are particularly vulnerable to sun-related complications. Sun exposure can trigger flare-ups, making these conditions worse. Sun protection

measures are crucial for managing and preventing these reactions.

6. Preventing Actinic Keratosis: Actinic keratosis is a precancerous skin condition often caused by sun exposure. Consistent sun protection can help prevent the development of actinic keratosis and lower the risk of it progressing into skin cancer.

7. Enhanced Skin Barrier Function: The sun can weaken the skin's natural barrier, making it more susceptible to irritants and allergens. Proper sun protection helps to maintain the integrity of the skin barrier, reducing the risk of conditions like contact dermatitis.

8. Lowered Risk of Photosensitivity Reactions: Some medications and skin

diseases make the skin more sensitive to sunlight, causing photosensitivity reactions. Protecting the skin from UV rays can minimize these reactions and the associated discomfort.

9. Preservation of Collagen and Elastin: UV radiation breaks down collagen and elastin fibers in the skin. Collagen and elastin are essential for skin firmness and elasticity. Sun protection helps preserve these structural components, preventing sagging and maintaining skin health.

Sun protection is paramount for the preservation of skin health and the prevention of various skin diseases. Prolonged sun exposure, especially without adequate protection, can have detrimental effects on the skin, from causing skin cancer to exacerbating existing skin conditions and promoting premature aging. Incorporating sun protection into your daily skincare routine is a simple yet powerful way to ensure your skin remains healthy, vibrant, and free from the many dangers posed by the sun's harmful rays. By using sunscreen, wearing protective clothing, seeking shade, and being mindful of sun exposure, you can significantly reduce the risk of skin diseases and maintain the health and beauty of your skin for years to come.

CHAPTER 6

NUTRITION AND YOUR SKIN

Nutrition plays a vital role in skin health, and the connection between what you eat and the development or management of skin diseases is profound. A well-balanced and nutrient-rich diet can promote skin health, while poor nutrition can exacerbate or even trigger various skin conditions. Here's a closer look at the relationship between nutrition and skin diseases:

1. Nutrients for Skin Health: Your skin requires a variety of nutrients to function optimally. These include vitamins (A, C, E), minerals (zinc, selenium), essential fatty acids (omega-3 and omega-6), and amino acids. These nutrients support the skin's natural repair and renewal processes, helping to keep it healthy.

2. Collagen Production: Collagen is a structural protein that gives the skin its firmness and elasticity. Vitamin C, found in many fruits and vegetables, is crucial for collagen production. Inadequate vitamin C intake can lead to sagging skin and delayed wound healing.

3. Antioxidants and Skin Protection: Antioxidants, such as vitamins A, C, and E, help protect the skin from damage caused by free radicals. Free radicals can accelerate the aging process and increase the risk of skin diseases, including skin cancer.

4. Omega-3 Fatty Acids: Omega-3 fatty acids, commonly found in fatty fish and flaxseeds, have anti-inflammatory properties that can help alleviate skin conditions like psoriasis and eczema. These healthy fats reduce redness, itching, and flakiness associated with these conditions.

5. Zinc for Wound Healing: Zinc is essential for the healing of wounds and the prevention of infections. In cases of skin diseases where the skin's integrity is compromised, such as open sores or ulcerations, adequate zinc intake is critical for proper healing.

6. Hydration through Diet: Proper hydration is essential for skin health. While drinking water is crucial, fruits and vegetables with high water content, like watermelon and cucumber, can contribute to skin hydration. Dehydrated skin is more prone to irritation and can exacerbate conditions like eczema and psoriasis.

7. Diet and Acne: There is a connection between diet and acne, particularly in the consumption of high-glycemic foods and dairy products. Diets high in sugar and dairy have been linked to increased acne severity. A diet rich in whole grains, fruits, and vegetables can help prevent acne breakouts.

8. Role of Probiotics: An imbalance of gut bacteria has been associated with skin conditions like acne, rosacea, and eczema. Consuming probiotic-rich foods, such as yogurt and kefir, can help balance the gut microbiome, potentially improving skin health.

9. Food Allergies and Skin Conditions: Food allergies or sensitivities can manifest on the skin as hives, eczema, or contact dermatitis. Identifying and avoiding trigger foods is essential in managing and preventing these skin reactions.

10. Skin Diseases and Malnutrition: In severe cases of malnutrition, the skin can become dry, scaly, and prone to infection. Conditions like kwashiorkor can result in a range of skin problems, underscoring the importance of proper nutrition.

In conclusion, nutrition plays a crucial role in skin health, and the relationship between diet and skin diseases is evident. A diet rich in a variety of nutrients, including vitamins, minerals, and healthy fats, can support skin health, promote healing, and reduce the risk of developing or exacerbating skin diseases. Conversely, poor dietary choices can lead to skin issues, such as acne, eczema, or premature aging. A balanced and nutrient-rich diet, combined with proper hydration, can be a powerful tool in preventing and managing skin diseases, ultimately leading to healthier and more radiant skin. It's essential to consult with a healthcare professional for personalized dietary advice, especially if you have specific skin concerns or conditions.

6.1 FOODS FOR HEALTHY SKIN

The hunt for healthy and radiant skin frequently begins with what you put on your plate. A balanced and nutrient-rich diet can do prodigies for your skin's health and appearance. Then are some foods that can contribute to healthy skin

1. Adipose Fish: Adipose fish like salmon, mackerel, and sardines are rich in omega- 3 adipose acids. These healthy fats help maintain the skin's lipid hedge, keeping it doused and precluding blankness. Omega- 3s also haveanti-inflammatory parcels that can palliate skin conditions like acne and psoriasis.

2. Avocado: Avocado is packed with healthy monounsaturated fats, vitamin

E, and antioxidants. These nutrients can help cover your skin from damage, promote its pliantness, and keep it looking immature.

3. Nuts and Seeds: Almonds, walnuts, sunflower seeds, and flaxseeds are excellent sources of vitamins E and C, as well as healthy fats. These nutrients combat oxidative stress and inflammation in the skin, reducing the threat of unseasonable aging.

4. Berries: Berries like blueberries, strawberries, and snorts are high in antioxidants, particularly vitaminC. Antioxidants help cover the skin from free radical damage and can promote a clear complexion.

5. Citrus Fruits: Citrus fruits, similar as oranges, failures, and grapefruits, are rich in vitamin C. This vitamin is essential for collagen product, which is pivotal for maintaining skin's firmness and precluding wrinkles.

6. Dark Leafy Greens: Spinach, kale, and Swiss chard are loaded with vitamins and minerals, including vitamin A, vitamin C, and folate. These lush flora promote skin form and help keep it doused .

7. Sweet Potatoes: Sweet potatoes are rich in beta- carotene, a precursor to vitaminA. Vitamin A is necessary for skin cell product and form. It can also help cover the skin from the sun's dangerous UV shafts.

8. Tomatoes: Tomatoes are a source of lycopene, an antioxidant that helps cover the skin from sun damage and may reduce the threat of sunburn. cuisine tomatoes in olive oil painting can enhance the immersion of lycopene.

9. Green Tea: Green tea contains polyphenols, which haveanti-inflammatory and antioxidant parcels. Drinking green tea can help cover the skin from damage and reduce the threat of skin conditions like acne and rosacea.

10. Yogurt: Yogurt is a good source of probiotics, which can promote a healthy gut microbiome. A balanced gut microbiome is linked to healthier skin, as an imbalance can lead to conditions like acne and eczema.

11. Water: While not a food, proper hydration is essential for healthy skin. Water keeps the skin doused and flushes out poisons. Dehydrated skin is more prone to blankness, vexation, and unseasonable aging.

12. Olive Oil: Olive oil painting is rich in healthy monounsaturated fats and antioxidants, which can help reduce inflammation and maintain skin's pliantness.

13. Carrots: Carrots are another source of beta- carotene, which not only supports skin health but can also give your skin a healthy gleam.

Incorporating these foods into your diet can go a long way in promoting healthy and beautiful skin. still, it's important to flash back that a balanced and varied diet is crucial. No single food can give all the nutrients your skin needs. also, it's essential to avoid or limit reused foods, inordinate sugar, and unhealthy fats, as these can contribute to skinissues.However, it's judicious to consult with a healthcare professional or a dermatologist for substantiated salutary guidance and skincare recommendations, If you have specific skin enterprises.

6.2 NUTRIENTS FOR SKIN HEALTH

The skin, our body's largest organ, plays a vital part in guarding us from the external terrain. To keep it performing optimally and looking its stylish, proper nutrition is essential. A well- balanced diet rich in specific nutrients can promote skin health and radiance. In this discussion, we'll explore the crucial nutrients that contribute to healthy skin and why they count.

1. Vitamin C: This antioxidant is a important supporter for skin health. It aids in collagen product, which helps maintain skin's firmness and pliantness. also, vitamin C combats the goods of UV radiation, which can accelerate the aging of the skin. Citrus fruits, strawberries, and bell peppers are excellent sources of this vitamin.

2. Vitamin E: Another antioxidant, vitamin E, protects the skin from damage caused by free revolutionaries. It also supports skin form and reduces inflammation. Almonds, spinach, and sunflower seeds are good sources of vitaminE.

3. Vitamin A: Vitamin A plays a pivotal part in skin cell product and form. It's essential for precluding dry, short skin and can also help reduce the appearance of wrinkles. Foods like sweet potatoes, carrots, and spinach are rich in vitaminA.

4. Omega- 3 Adipose Acids: These healthy fats help maintain the skin's lipid hedge, which keeps it doused and prevents blankness. Omega- 3s are set up in adipose fish like salmon, flaxseeds, and walnuts.

5. Zinc This mineral supports: the skin's natural mending process and helps control inflammation. It's especially salutary for individualities with acne-prone skin. Foods like spare flesh, nuts, and whole grains are good sources of zinc.

6. Collagen: Collagen is a protein that provides structure to the skin. While not attained directly from food, collagen product can be stimulated by consuming vitamin C-rich foods and amino acids set up in protein sources.

7. Hydration: While not a nutrient, proper hydration is abecedarian for skin health. Water keeps the skin moisturized, which is essential for a healthy complexion. Dehumidification can lead to blankness, flakiness, and an increased threat of wrinkles.

8. Antioxidants: A diet rich in antioxidants, similar as those set up in fruits and vegetables, can cover the skin from damage and inflammation. Berries, green tea, and dark chocolate are excellent sources.

9. Selenium: Selenium is a mineral that can help cover the skin from sun damage and skin cancer. It's set up in foods like Brazil nuts, whole wheat chuck, and lemon.

10. Probiotics: Gut health is linked to skin health, and probiotics can help maintain a balanced gut microbiome. A healthy gut can reduce inflammation and skin conditions like acne. Yogurt, kefir, and kimchi are sources of probiotics. It's important to note that while these nutrients play a significant part in skin health, they're most effective when part of a well- rounded, balanced diet. also, individual skin types and conditions can impact which nutrients are most salutary. Consultation with a healthcare professional or dermatologist can give substantiated guidance.   In conclusion, a diet rich in specific nutrients, including vitamins C and E, omega- 3 adipose acids, and antioxidants, is pivotal for maintaining healthy and vibrant skin.

These nutrients give protection against environmental damage, support the skin's structure, and aid in form and rejuvenescence. Coupled with proper hydration and a well- rounded diet, these rudiments are the foundation for glowing and immature skin.

CHAPTER 7

LIFESTYLE FACTORS AND SKIN CARE

Life Factors and Skin Care in Dealing with Skin conditions

Skin conditions can have a profound impact on a person's quality of life. Conditions similar as acne, eczema, psoriasis, and skin cancer can beget physical discomfort, emotional torture, and social insulation. While medical treatments play a vital part in managing these conditions, life factors and proper skin care are inversely important in precluding and managing skin conditions.

** **Diet and Nutrition** ** A well-balanced diet plays a pivotal part in maintaining healthy skin. Nutrients similar as vitamins A, C, and E, along with omega- 3 adipose acids, are known to promote skin health. These factors help cover the skin from damage caused by free revolutionaries, support collagen product, and maintain proper hydration. also, staying adequately doused is essential for precluding dry skin and promoting overall skin health.

** **Sun Protection** ** Dragged exposure to the sun's dangerous ultraviolet(UV) shafts is a significant factor in the development of skin conditions, including skin cancer. Sunscreen with a high SPF standing should be an integral part of your diurnal skincare routine. Avoiding sun exposure during peak hours and wearing defensive apparel, similar as wide-brimmed headdresses and sunglasses, are also important for skin protection.

Smoking and Alcohol Consumption Smoking and inordinate alcohol consumption can have mischievous goods on the skin. Smoking reduces blood inflow to the skin, leading to unseasonable aging and adding the threat of skin cancer. Alcohol dehydrates the skin, making it more prone to damage. Quitting smoking and moderating alcohol input can significantly ameliorate skin health.

Stress operation habitual stress can spark or complicate skin conditions similar as acne and psoriasis. Stress increases inflammation throughout the body, including the skin. enforcing stress- reduction ways like contemplation, yoga, and exercise can help manage these conditions.

** **Hygiene Practices** ** Maintaining good hygiene is abecedarian in precluding skin conditions. Regularly washing the face and body with mild, pH- balanced cleaners helps remove dirt, redundant oil painting, and bacteria. still, overwashing or using harsh detergents can lead to blankness and vexation. Chancing the right balance is essential.

** **Moisturizing** ** Keeping the skin adequately moisturized is essential for maintaining its natural hedge function. People with conditions like eczema and psoriasis benefit from diurnal moisturizing to help flare- ups. Using scent-free, hypoallergenic moisturizers can help minimize skin vexation.

 ** **Avoiding annoyances** ** relating and avoiding implicit annoyances is pivotal for individualities with sensitive skin or skin conditions. This includes choosing hypoallergenic products and avoiding known triggers, similar as certain cosmetics or harsh cleansers.

 ** **Regular Check- ups** ** Routine skin examinations by a dermatologist are essential for early discovery of skin conditions, especially skin cancer. Detecting and treating skin conditions in their early stages can greatly ameliorate the chances of successful operation.

In conclusion, life factors and proper skin care are integral in dealing with skin conditions. A holistic approach to skin health encompasses diet, sun protection, stress operation, and hygiene practices. By espousing these habits, individualities can't only help numerous skin conditions but also ameliorate their overall quality of life. It's important to flash back that while life changes can be effective in managing and precluding skin conditions, medical advice and treatment from a dermatologist should be sought when necessary to insure the stylish possible outgrowth.

7.1 STRESS MANAGEMENT

The intricate connection between stress and skin health is a well- established fact. In dealing with skin conditions, effective stress operation plays a vital part in both forestallment and treatment. Stress not only exacerbates colorful skin conditions but can also be a primary detector for their onset. Understanding this relationship and enforcing stress operation strategies is pivotal for maintaining healthy skin.

 ** **Stress and Skin Health** ** When the body is under stress, it releases a hormone called cortisol. Elevated cortisol situations can lead to inflammation and increased oil painting product in the skin, making it more susceptible to conditions like acne, psoriasis, and eczema. Stress can also decelerate down the skin's natural mending processes, leading to longer recovery times for injuries, blisters, and skin infections.

** **Mind- Body Connection** ** The mind- body connection is important, and it directly affects skin health. Emotional stress can manifest physically on the skin, leading to symptoms similar as hives, rashes, and indeed aggravating habitual skin conditions. Stress can also lead to the bad habit of skin- selecting, which can further worsen being skin issues.

** **Stress Reduction ways** **
Managing stress effectively can have a significant positive impact on skin

conditions. Then are some stress reduction ways that can help

1. ** Contemplation and awareness ** Meditation and awareness practices can calm the mind and reduce stress. These ways help individualities come more apprehensive of their studies and feelings, allowing them to respond to stressors more calmly.

2. ** Yoga ** Yoga combines physical postures, breathing exercises, and contemplation to reduce stress and ameliorate overall well- being. Regular practice can help control stress- related skin symptoms.

3. ** Exercise ** Regular physical exertion releases endorphins, which are natural mood boosters. Exercise also

improves blood rotation, which is salutary for skin health. Engaging in conditioning you enjoy, like walking, swimming, or dancing, can be both fun and stress- reducing.

4. ** Healthy Diet ** A balanced diet that includes fruits, vegetables, and whole grains provides the body with essential nutrients. Avoiding inordinate caffeine, sugar, and reused foods can help regulate blood sugar situations and reduce skin inflammation.

5. ** Acceptable Sleep ** Quality sleep is pivotal for managing stress and promoting skin health. Aim for 7- 9 hours of peaceful sleep each night to allow your skin to repair and regenerate.

6. ** Social Support ** Talking to musketeers, family, or a therapist can be an effective way to manage with stress. participating your enterprises and passions can palliate emotional burdens and reduce stress- related skin symptoms.

7. ** Relaxation ways ** ways like deep breathing exercises, progressive muscle relaxation, and aromatherapy can help you relax and reduce stress situations.

** Professional Help ** In some cases, dealing with stress on your own may not beenough.However, seeking help from a internal health professional or therapist can give precious guidance and support, If stress is significantly impacting your skin health. They can help you develop managing strategies and address the root causes of your stress.

In conclusion, stress operation is a critical aspect of dealing with skin conditions. The mind- body connection is a important one, and stress can significantly impact the onset and exacerbation of colorful skin conditions. By enforcing stress reduction ways, individualities can't only ameliorate their overall well- being but also manage and help skin conditions more effectively. Flash back that while stress operation is important, consulting with a dermatologist for medical treatment and guidance is inversely essential in the operation of specific skin conditions.

7.2 SLEEP AND SKIN REGENERATION

The significance of sleep in maintaining overall health can not be exaggerated, and it holds particular significance in the environment of skin health. Sleep is a critical time for skin rejuvenescence and form, making it a vital element in the forestallment and operation of skin conditions. Understanding the relationship between sleep and skin can lead to further effective strategies for dealing with colorful skin conditions.

Skin rejuvenescence During Sleep: While we sleep, the body undergoes multitudinous restorative processes, including skin rejuvenescence. The most significant exertion takes place during the deeper stages of sleep, especially rapid-fire eye movement(REM) sleep. During these phases, the body's product of growth hormone and melatonin increases. Growth hormone stimulates the product of collagen, the protein that provides structure and pliantness to the skin. Melatonin, in addition to regulating the sleep- wake cycle, acts as an antioxidant, guarding the skin from oxidative stress.

The Impact of Sleep Deprivation:
When individualities constantly witness sleep privation, their bodies don't have sufficient time to complete the necessary skin form processes. This can affect in colorful adverse goods on the skin, including

1. Accelerated Aging: habitual sleep privation can lead to unseasonable aging of the skin, characterized by the development of wrinkles, fine lines, and a loss of skin pliantness.

2. Blankness and Dullness: Lack of sleep can vitiate the skin's capability to retain humidity, leading to blankness and dullness. It can also worsen being skin conditions like eczema and psoriasis.

3. Acne and flights: Sleep privation can increase inflammation in the body, which can complicate conditions like acne. It can also affect the skin's capability to heal mars, leading to dragged flights.

4. Bloodied Wound Healing:

Acceptable sleep is pivotal for effective crack mending. Sleep- deprived individualities may witness delayed mending of cuts, becks
, and other skin injuries.

STRATEGIES FOR ADVANCED SLEEP AND SKIN HEALTH:

To promote skin rejuvenescence and overall skin health, it's essential to prioritize good sleep hygiene. Then are some strategies

1. Establish a Routine: Aim for a harmonious sleep schedule, going to bed and waking up at the same times each day.

2. Produce a Comfortable Sleep terrain: insure that your sleep terrain is conducive to rest. This includes a comfortable mattress and pillow, a cool room, and minimum exposure to light and noise.

3. Limit Screen Time: The blue light emitted by defenses can disrupt sleep. Steer clear of stimulating activities at least an hour before bedtime.

4. Relaxation ways: Engage in relaxation conditioning before bed, similar as reading, gentle stretching, or contemplation.

5. Moderate Caffeine and Alcohol: Both caffeine and alcohol can intrude with sleep quality. Have a consumption Limit in the evenings especially.

6. Manage Stress: Stress can significantly impact sleep quality. Employ stress operation ways, similar as deep breathing exercises or awareness, to reduce stress situations.

7. Physical exertion: Regular exercise can promote better sleep, but avoid violent exercises close to bedtime.

Sleep is a pivotal factor in skin rejuvenescence and plays a significant part in dealing with skin conditions. Acceptable, high- quality sleep allows the body to perform essential skin form and rejuvenescence processes, which can prop in the forestallment and operation of colorful skin conditions. By prioritizing good sleep hygiene and seeking professional advice when necessary, individualities can ameliorate their skin health and overall well- being.

CHAPTER 8

COMMON SKIN CONDITIONS

Understanding common skin conditions is essential for proper forestallment, opinion, and treatment. Then, we'll claw into some of the most current skin conditions and explore how they can be managed.

1. Acne: Acne is one of the most common skin conditions, affecting individualities of all periods. It generally arises when hair follicles come congested with oil painting and dead skin cells. Acne can manifest as blackheads, papules, or painful excrescencies. Proper sanctification, topical treatments, and occasionally tradition specifics are used to manage acne.

2. Eczema(Dermatitis): Eczema is a group of skin conditions characterized by inflammation, greenishness, and itchiness. It frequently presents with dry, scaled patches. While the exact cause of eczema isn't completely understood, it's believed to involve a combination of inheritable and environmental factors. Managing eczema frequently involves moisturizing, avoiding triggers, and using topical corticosteroids.

3. Psoriasis: Psoriasis is a habitual autoimmune skin complaint that results in the rapid-fire buildup of skin cells. This leads to scaling, inflammation, and greenishness. Psoriasis can affect any part of the body and may have a inheritable element. operation includes topical treatments, light remedy, and systemic specifics.

4. Rosacea: Rosacea is a habitual skin condition that primarily affects the face. It leads to greenishness, visible blood vessels, and, in some cases, acne-suchlike papules. While the cause of rosacea is unclear, triggers similar as racy foods, alcohol, and sun exposure can complicate the condition. Topical and oral specifics are used to manage rosacea.

5. Skin Cancer: Skin cancer, including carcinoma, rudimentary cell melanoma, and scaled cell melanoma, is a significant concern. Ultraviolet(UV) radiation from the sun and tanning beds is a primary threat factor. Prevention involves sun protection, including sunscreen and defensive apparel. Beforehand discovery and surgical junking of cancerous growths are crucial to effective treatment.

6. Hives(Urticaria): Hives are red, itchy welts that can appear suddenly and vanish within hours. They're frequently touched off by disinclinations or stress. Antihistamines can help relieve the symptoms of hives, and relating and avoiding triggers is essential.

7. Fungal Infections: Fungal infections like athlete's bottom and ringworm are common skin conditions caused by colorful fungi. They're generally treated with topical antifungal creams or oral specifics in severe cases.

8. Contact Dermatitis: Contact dermatitis is an antipathetic response or vexation of the skin when exposed to specific substances, similar as bane ivy, spices, or chemicals. Avoiding the annoyances or allergens is the primary treatment, along with topical corticosteroids.

9. Knobs: Knobs are caused by the mortal papillomavirus(HPV) and can appear on any part of the body. They're generally inoffensive but can be bothersome. Treatment options include untoward results, tradition specifics, and in- office procedures like cryotherapy.

10. Herpes: Herpes infections, caused by the herpes simplex contagion(HSV), can lead to oral herpes(cold blisters) and genital herpes. Antiviral specifics can help manage outbreaks and reduce their inflexibility.

Effective operation of common skin conditions frequently involves a combination of life changes, topical treatments, and, in some cases, specifics. It's pivotal to consult a dermatologist or healthcare professional for a proper opinion and treatment plan acclimatized to the specific skin condition. also, maintaining a healthy life, rehearsing good skin hygiene, and guarding the skin from environmental factors like UV radiation are essential for overall skin health and the forestallment of skin conditions.

8.1 ACNE MANAGEMENT

Acne, a common skin condition that affects people of all periods, can be both physically and emotionally distressing. While there's no bone

- size- fits- all result, effective acne operation involves a combination of skincare practices, life adaptations, and, in some cases, medical interventions. Then, we explore colorful strategies to help you achieve clearer and healthier skin.

1. Gentle Cleansing: Start with a gentle sanctification routine. Use a mild, pH-balanced cleaner to remove redundant oil painting, dirt, and dead skin cells without causing vexation. Avoid harsh scrubbing, as it can complicate acne.

2. Avoid Overwashing: While it's important to keep your skin clean, overwashing can strip your skin of its natural canvases , leading to blankness and potentially worsening acne. doubly-diurnal sanctification is generally sufficient.

3. Non-comedogenic Products: Choose skincare and makeup products labeled as"non-comedogenic." These are formulated to avoid congesting pores, reducing the threat of acne flights.

4. Moisturize: Contrary to common belief, indeed if you have acne-prone skin, moisturizing is pivotal. Use a featherlight, oil painting-free, ornon-comedogenic moisturizer to maintain skin hydration without causing flights.

5. Sun Protection: cover your skin from the sun by using a broad- diapason sunscreen with at least SPF 30. Some acne specifics can make the skin more sensitive to sun, so sun protection is essential.

6. Acne- fighting constituents: Look for products containing effective acne- fighting constituents like benzoyl peroxide, salicylic acid, or nascence hydroxy acids(AHAs). These approaches can aid in diminishing inflammation and clearing blocked pores.

7. Avoid Picking and Squeezing: defying the appetite to pick or squeeze acne mars is pivotal. Doing so can lead to scarring, infections, and worsened flights.

8. Diet and Nutrition: Some studies suggest a link between diet and acne. While further exploration is demanded, a healthy diet rich in fruits, vegetables, whole grains, and spare proteins can support overall skin health.

9. Stress operation: High stress situations can complicate acne. Incorporate stress- reduction ways similar as contemplation, yoga, or deep breathing exercises into your diurnal routine.

10. Avoid Alarms: Identify and avoid implicit triggers that worsen your acne. This can encompass various factors such as specific dietary choices, the use of particular cosmetics, or exposure to certain environmental elements.

Professional Care: In some cases, untoward products may not be enough to manage acne. Consider seeking professional help from a dermatologist who can give a individualized treatment plan. Common medical treatments for acne include

Tradition Topicals: Dermatologists can define stronger topical treatments, similar as retinoids or antibiotics, to target more severe acne.

Oral specifics: Antibiotics and hormonal specifics may be recommended for certain types of acne, particularly when untoward treatments are ineffective.

Isotretinoin: For severe, patient acne that does not respond to other treatments, isotretinoin, a important drug, may be specified. It has the eventuality for side goods and requires careful monitoring.

Procedures: In- office procedures like chemical peels, microdermabrasion, or ray remedy can be used to treat acne and acne scars.

Life Changes: A dermatologist can also give guidance on life adaptations that may ameliorate your skin health, similar as salutary variations or recommendations for managing stress.

Effective acne operation takes time and tolerance. It's essential to stick with your skincare routine and any prescribed treatments constantly. Results may not be immediate, but with continuity, you can achieve clearer, healthier skin. Flash back that everyone's skin is unique, so what works for one person may not work for another. Consulting a dermatologist is an excellent step if you are floundering to manage your acne effectively. They can give expert guidance and knitter a treatment plan to your specific requirements.

8.2 ECZEMA, DERMATITIS AND PSORIASIS

Eczema and psoriasis are habitual skin conditions that affect millions of individualities worldwide. While they partake some parallels in their symptoms, causes, and treatment approaches, they're distinct conditions with unique characteristics. This comprehensive examination will claw into the crucial aspects of eczema and psoriasis, exploring their causes, symptoms, opinion, and available treatments.

ECZEMA(DERMATITIS)

Eczema, also known as dermatitis, is a common skin condition characterized by inflammation, greenishness, and itching.

It can manifest as dry, scaled patches on the skin and can affect individualities of all periods, including babies. Eczema is frequently used as a general term for colorful forms of dermatitis, with atopic dermatitis being the most common. Let's explore the crucial aspects of eczema

Causes

The exact cause of eczema isn't entirely understood, but it's believed to affect from a combination of inheritable and environmental factors. individualities with a family history of eczema or other antipathetic conditions like asthma or hay fever may be more prone to developing it. Environmental factors, similar as exposure to annoyances or allergens, can spark or worsen eczema.

Symptoms

Eczema generally presents as red, itchy, and inflamed skin. The inflexibility of symptoms can vary, with some individualities passing only mild itching and blankness, while others may have violent itching and wide rashes. The skin may come thickened or develop painful cracks, especially in severe cases. Common areas affected by eczema include the face, neck, hands, and inner crimps of the elbows and knees.

Opinion

Diagnosing eczema generally involves a physical examination by a dermatologist or healthcare provider. They will assess the appearance of the skin, interrogate about particular or family history of skin conditions, disinclinations, and any known triggers.

In some cases, a patch test may be performed to identify specific allergens that complicate the condition.

Treatment

Eczema operation focuses on symptom relief, reducing inflammation, and precluding flare- ups. Some common approaches include

Topical Steroids: Topical corticosteroids are frequently specified to reduce inflammation and itching. They come in colorful strengths, and the choice depends on the inflexibility of the condition.

Emollients and Moisturizers: Regular use of emollients and moisturizers helps maintain skin hydration, reducing blankness and itchiness.

Avoiding Triggers: relating and avoiding triggers similar as certain detergents, cleansers, allergens, and annoyances is essential in managing eczema.

Antihistamines: In cases of severe itching, antihistamines may be recommended to palliate discomfort.

Phototherapy: In some cases, exposure to ultraviolet(UV) light, under controlled conditions, can help ameliorate symptoms.

PSORIASIS

Psoriasis is a habitual autoimmune skin complaint characterized by the rapid-fire overproduction of skin cells. The redundant skin cells accumulate on the face, leading to the conformation of thick, red, scaled pillars. Psoriasis is known for its distinct appearance and is associated with a range of implicit complications, including psoriatic arthritis. Then are the crucial aspects of psoriasis

Causes

The precise cause of psoriasis isn't completely understood, but it's believed to involve an abnormal vulnerable response. Genetics plays a significant part, as individualities with a family history of psoriasis are at advanced threat. External factors, similar as infections, injuries, or stress, can spark or complicate psoriasis in genetically fitted individualities.

Symptoms

Psoriasis presents with red, raised, scaled patches of skin, which can appear anywhere on the body. The inflexibility and position of these pillars can vary extensively among individualities. Some may have a many small, localized areas of involvement, while others may witness wide content. Psoriasis is frequently associated with itching, burning, or discomfort, and it can affect the nails and joints, leading to nail and joint problems in some cases.

Opinion

Diagnosing psoriasis is generally grounded on a physical examination of the skin and nails by a dermatologist. There are different types of psoriasis, including shrine psoriasis(the most common form), guttate psoriasis, pustular psoriasis, and others, each with its distinctive features. Necropsies or fresh tests are occasionally demanded for a precise opinion.

Treatment

Psoriasis treatment aims to manage symptoms, control the rate of skin cell development, and ameliorate overall quality of life. colorful approaches include

Topical Treatments: These include topical corticosteroids, vitamin D analogs, and retinoids. These are applied directly to affected areas.

Systemic specifics: For more severe cases, oral or fitted specifics, similar as biologics, immunosuppressants, or methotrexate, may be specified to control inflammation and slow skin cell product.

Phototherapy: Light remedy, which involves exposure to UVB light, is an effective treatment for psoriasis.

Lifestyle and Diet: Certain life changes, similar as managing stress, quitting smoking, and maintaining a healthy weight, can help manage psoriasis. Some individualities may also profit from salutary variations, similar as avoiding detector foods or alcohol.

Crucial Differences

While eczema and psoriasis partake some parallels, they've identifying characteristics

Appearance: Eczema generally presents as red, inflamed, itchy patches that may be dry and scaled, while psoriasis is characterized by thick, raised, scaled pillars.

Causes: Eczema frequently has antipathetic or irritant triggers, while psoriasis is an autoimmune condition.

Age of Onset: Eczema can affect individualities of all periods, including babies, while psoriasis generally develops in majority.

Treatment Approaches: Treatment for eczema primarily focuses on symptom relief and detector avoidance, while psoriasis treatments frequently target vulnerable responses and skin cell development.

In conclusion, eczema and psoriasis are two current skin conditions with distinct characteristics, causes, and treatment approaches. While both can beget significant discomfort and affect an existent's quality of life, they can be managed effectively with proper care and medicalguidance.However, seeking the moxie of a dermatologist is essential for accurate opinion and substantiated treatment, If you suspect you have eczema or psoriasis. With the right operation strategies, individualities with these conditions can achieve better control of their symptoms and enjoy healthier skin.

CHAPTER 9

DIY SKIN CARE REMEDIES

When dealing with skin diseases, many individuals turn to do-it-yourself (DIY) skin care remedies to complement their treatment regimens. These natural approaches often offer gentler, cost-effective solutions for various skin conditions. While DIY remedies may not replace medical treatments, they can provide added relief and support. Here are some popular DIY skin care remedies for common skin issues:

1. Honey for Acne: Honey is a natural antimicrobial and anti-inflammatory agent. Applying raw, organic honey to acne-prone areas can help reduce inflammation, kill bacteria, and promote wound healing. As a mask or spot treatment, it can be effective in managing acne symptoms.

2. Oatmeal for Eczema: Oatmeal baths are a tried-and-true remedy for soothing the itching and inflammation associated with eczema. Simply grind oatmeal into a fine powder and add it to a warm bath. The colloidal oatmeal will relieve discomfort and moisturize the skin.

3. Aloe Vera for Sunburn: Aloe vera is renowned for its soothing and cooling properties. The gel extracted from aloe leaves can be applied directly to sunburned skin to alleviate pain and redness. Its natural anti-inflammatory properties aid in the healing process.

4. Coconut Oil for Psoriasis: Coconut oil is a natural moisturizer that can help soothe the scaling and redness associated with psoriasis. Applying extra-virgin coconut oil to affected areas can provide relief from dryness and discomfort.

5. Green Tea for Rosacea: Green tea contains antioxidants and anti-inflammatory compounds that can help reduce the redness and inflammation associated with rosacea. After brewing and cooling green tea, applying it to the affected area using a cotton ball can offer relief.

6. Apple Cider Vinegar for Skin Tags: While it's crucial to consult a dermatologist for proper diagnosis and removal, some people use apple cider vinegar as a natural remedy for skin tags. Applying a small amount with a cotton ball may cause the skin tag to fall off over time.

7. Lemon Juice for Hyperpigmentation: Lemon juice contains natural citric acid, which can help lighten dark spots and hyperpigmentation. Dilute lemon juice with water and apply it to affected areas for a few minutes before rinsing. Be cautious, as lemon juice can make your skin more sensitive to sunlight, so wear sunscreen during the day.

8. Baking Soda for Exfoliation: A simple mixture of baking soda and water can be used as a gentle exfoliant to remove dead skin cells, making it a cost-effective way to improve skin texture. Do not use it on broken skin.

It's essential to keep in mind that DIY skin care remedies may not be suitable for every skin type or condition. Allergic reactions, irritation, or worsening of the condition can occur if a remedy isn't appropriate for your specific situation. Before trying any DIY remedies, consult a dermatologist or healthcare professional for guidance. They can help you identify the best approach for your skin type and condition, ensuring that the remedies you choose are safe and effective.

DIY skin care remedies can be a beneficial addition to your skincare routine, offering natural alternatives for managing common skin issues. While they may not replace medical treatments entirely, these remedies can provide comfort and relief, supporting your journey toward healthier, clearer skin.

9.1 NATURAL INGREDIENTS FOR SKIN

The world of skincare has seen a resurgence in the use of natural ingredients for managing various skin conditions and promoting overall skin health. These natural remedies, often derived from plants, fruits, and other sources, offer a holistic approach to treating skin diseases. Let's explore some of the most popular natural ingredients and their potential benefits in addressing skin issues:

1. **Aloe Vera:** Aloe vera is a renowned natural ingredient with multiple benefits for the skin. It is known for its soothing properties, making it effective in treating sunburns, irritations, and minor burns.

Aloe vera's natural gel can help reduce inflammation and promote healing.

2. Tea Tree Oil: Derived from the leaves of the tea tree, this essential oil has powerful antibacterial and anti-inflammatory properties. It's commonly used to treat acne and fungal skin infections. You can apply diluted tea tree oil directly to the affected skin areas for targeted relief.

3. Coconut Oil: Coconut oil is a natural moisturizer rich in fatty acids. It's beneficial for dry skin and conditions like eczema and psoriasis. Applying extra-virgin coconut oil to the skin helps lock in moisture and reduce irritation.

4. Honey: Raw honey is a natural humectant, meaning it helps retain moisture in the skin. It's also antimicrobial, making it effective in treating acne and minor wounds. Honey can be used as a spot treatment or incorporated into masks.

5. Chamomile: Chamomile has anti-inflammatory and antioxidant properties, making it beneficial for soothing irritated skin. Chamomile tea bags can be steeped and used as a compress for skin conditions like eczema or rosacea.

6. Turmeric: Known for its anti-inflammatory properties, turmeric can help reduce redness and swelling. Turmeric paste, made from turmeric powder and water, can be applied to areas affected by conditions like psoriasis or acne.

7. Oatmeal: Oatmeal is a natural exfoliant and skin soother. Ground oatmeal can be used in bath soaks to relieve itching and inflammation in conditions such as eczema and dermatitis.

8. Green Tea: Green tea is rich in antioxidants that help protect the skin from damage caused by free radicals. Topical application or the use of skincare products containing green tea extracts can benefit various skin conditions.

9. Cucumber: Cucumber has a high water content and contains anti-inflammatory compounds. Slices of cucumber can be placed on the eyes to reduce puffiness, and cucumber puree can be applied as a cooling mask for sensitive or irritated skin.

10. Witch Hazel: Witch hazel is a natural astringent and anti-inflammatory agent. It's often used to soothe and tone the skin, making it beneficial for conditions like acne and eczema.

While these natural ingredients have the potential to benefit skin health and manage certain skin diseases, it's essential to remember that individual responses can vary. Patch tests are often recommended, especially for those with sensitive skin, to ensure there are no adverse reactions. Additionally, these natural remedies may complement medical treatments but should not replace professional guidance for severe or persistent skin conditions. Consulting a dermatologist for a precise diagnosis and treatment plan is crucial for comprehensive skin health management.

By incorporating natural ingredients into your skincare routine, you can explore gentler, more holistic approaches to managing common skin issues and maintaining healthy, radiant skin.

9.2 HOMEMADE SKIN CARE RECIPES

Homemade skin care recipes offer a natural and cost-effective way to address various skin diseases and promote healthier skin. These DIY remedies often utilize common kitchen ingredients and can be tailored to suit individual skin types and conditions. Here, we explore a selection of homemade skin care recipes that can be beneficial in managing skin diseases.

1. Oatmeal Face Mask for Eczema:
- Ingredients: Rolled oats, honey, plain yogurt
- Method: Blend a small amount of rolled oats into a fine powder. Mix with honey and yogurt to create a paste. Apply the

mask to affected areas and leave it on for 15-20 minutes before rinsing with warm water. This soothing mask can relieve itching and inflammation associated with eczema.

2. Turmeric and Honey Paste for Acne:

- Ingredients: Turmeric powder, honey
- Method: Combine turmeric powder and honey to create a thick paste. Apply it to acne-prone areas and leave it on for 10-15 minutes. Turmeric's anti-inflammatory and antibacterial properties, along with honey's soothing effects, can help manage acne breakouts.

3. Green Tea Toner for Rosacea:

- Ingredients: Green tea bag, boiling water

- Method: Steep a green tea bag in boiling water, allow it to cool, and then transfer it to a spray bottle. Use the green tea toner to mist the face or apply it with a cotton pad. The antioxidants in green tea can help reduce redness and inflammation associated with rosacea.

4. Honey and Cinnamon Spot Treatment for Acne:

- Ingredients: Honey, cinnamon powder
- Method: Mix honey and cinnamon powder to create a paste. Apply a small amount to individual acne spots and leave it on for 15-20 minutes. This spot treatment harnesses the antimicrobial properties of honey and the anti-inflammatory effects of cinnamon.

5. Avocado and Honey Moisturizing Mask for Dry Skin:

- Ingredients: Ripe avocado, honey
- Method: Mash a ripe avocado and mix it with honey to form a smooth paste. Apply the mask to dry skin areas and leave it on for 15-20 minutes. Avocado's natural oils and honey's moisturizing properties work together to hydrate and soothe dry skin.

6. Cucumber and Aloe Vera Gel for Sunburn:

- Ingredients: Cucumber, aloe vera gel
- **Method:** Blend a cucumber into a puree and mix it with aloe vera gel. Apply this cooling mixture to sunburned areas for instant relief. The soothing properties of cucumber and aloe vera can help reduce redness and discomfort.

Homemade skin care recipes offer a natural and often gentler approach to managing skin diseases. While these remedies can be beneficial for common skin issues, it's essential to remember that individual responses may vary. Patch testing is recommended, especially for sensitive skin, to ensure there are no adverse reactions.

Moreover, these DIY remedies are most effective when used as complementary treatments, not as substitutes for professional guidance. Dermatologists can provide precise diagnoses and treatment plans for severe or persistent skin conditions. By incorporating homemade skin care recipes into your skincare routine, you can explore natural solutions that suit your specific skin needs and contribute to healthier, more radiant skin.

CHAPTER 10

ADVANCED SKIN CARE TECHNIQUES

Advanced skin care techniques have revolutionized the management of skin diseases, offering more effective and precise solutions for a wide range of dermatological conditions. These innovative approaches incorporate cutting-edge technologies, research-based treatments, and a deeper understanding of skin biology. Let's explore some of the advanced techniques that are transforming the field of dermatology in dealing with skin diseases.

1. Biologics for Psoriasis:

Biologics are a class of medications developed to target the specific immune system processes responsible for psoriasis. These advanced treatments, which are typically administered by injection, are highly effective in managing the disease. Biologics have transformed the lives of many psoriasis patients by providing long-lasting relief and even complete clearance of symptoms.

2. Photodynamic Therapy (PDT) for Actinic Keratosis:

PDT is a technique used to treat actinic keratosis, which are precancerous skin lesions caused by sun exposure. PDT involves the application of a photosensitizing agent to the affected area, followed by exposure to a specific type of light. The light activates the photosensitizing agent, destroying the precancerous cells.

3. Mohs Micrographic Surgery for Skin Cancer:

Mohs surgery is an advanced technique for treating skin cancer, particularly basal cell carcinoma and squamous cell carcinoma. It involves the removal of the tumor layer by layer while examining each layer under a microscope until no cancerous cells remain. This precise method offers an extremely high cure rate and minimizes damage to healthy tissue.

4. Fractional Laser Resurfacing for Scarring:

Fractional laser resurfacing is used to treat acne scars and other types of scarring. It works by creating controlled micro-injuries in the skin, stimulating collagen production and improving skin texture. This advanced technology offers more predictable and less invasive results compared to traditional laser resurfacing.

5. Platelet-Rich Plasma (PRP) for Hair Loss and Skin Rejuvenation:

PRP therapy involves drawing a patient's blood, processing it to concentrate platelets, and then injecting the platelet-rich plasma into the skin or scalp. PRP has shown promise in promoting hair regrowth in cases of androgenetic alopecia and rejuvenating the skin for a more youthful appearance.

6. Cryotherapy for Warts and Skin Lesions:

Cryotherapy uses extremely cold temperatures to freeze and remove skin lesions such as warts. Liquid nitrogen is commonly used in this procedure, which is a quick and effective way to treat various dermatological conditions.

7. Targeted Phototherapy for Vitiligo:
Vitiligo is a challenging skin condition characterized by the loss of pigment. Targeted phototherapy involves delivering narrowband UVB light to the depigmented areas, stimulating melanocyte production. This advanced technique can help repigment the skin and improve the appearance of vitiligo.

8. Laser and Light Therapies for Acne and Rosacea:
Lasers and intense pulsed light (IPL) therapies are advanced methods for

treating acne and rosacea. They target the underlying causes of these conditions, such as excess sebum production and blood vessel dilation, leading to significant symptom reduction.

9. Microbiome-based Skin Care:
Recent research has highlighted the role of the skin microbiome in maintaining skin health. Advanced skin care products now incorporate microbiome-friendly ingredients to balance and support the skin's natural microbial ecosystem, potentially aiding in conditions like acne and eczema.

These advanced skin care techniques have revolutionized the field of dermatology, offering innovative solutions for various skin diseases.

While these treatments can provide remarkable results, it's crucial to consult a dermatologist to determine the most appropriate and effective approach for your specific condition. Dermatologists are uniquely trained to diagnose, treat, and provide personalized recommendations to address skin diseases, ensuring the best possible outcomes and the health of your skin.

10.1 PROFESSIONAL TREATMENTS

Skin diseases can be challenging to manage, and professional treatments offer effective solutions for many of these conditions. Dermatologists and healthcare professionals are trained to diagnose, treat, and provide specialized care for various skin disorders. Here are some of the professional treatments commonly used to address skin diseases:

1. Topical Medications: Dermatologists often prescribe topical medications for treating skin conditions. These may include corticosteroids to reduce inflammation, antibiotics for bacterial infections, or retinoids to address acne and psoriasis. These medications are applied directly to the skin and can be tailored to the specific needs of each patient.

2. Oral Medications: In some cases, oral medications are necessary for more severe skin diseases. Antibiotics are commonly used to treat conditions like severe acne, while immunosuppressants or systemic retinoids may be prescribed for diseases like psoriasis or eczema.

3. Light and Laser Therapies: Dermatologists utilize various light-based treatments to manage skin diseases. Photodynamic therapy (PDT) is used for actinic keratosis and certain types of skin cancer. Laser therapy can be effective for conditions such as rosacea, acne, and scars. Intense pulsed light (IPL) is another treatment option for vascular and pigment-related skin conditions.

4. Cryotherapy: Cryotherapy involves the use of extremely cold temperatures to freeze and remove skin lesions such as warts, actinic keratosis, and skin tags. Liquid nitrogen is commonly used in this procedure, which is a quick and effective way to treat various dermatological conditions.

5. Biologic Therapies: Biologics are advanced treatments often used to manage autoimmune skin diseases like psoriasis. These medications target specific immune system processes responsible for the disease, providing significant symptom relief.

6. Injectable Treatments: Cosmetic injectables such as botulinum toxin (Botox) and dermal fillers are used for a range of dermatological issues. Botox can reduce the appearance of wrinkles and fine lines, while dermal fillers can address volume loss, scars, and uneven skin texture.

7. Mohs Micrographic Surgery: Mohs surgery is a specialized procedure for skin cancer, particularly basal cell carcinoma and squamous cell carcinoma. It involves the removal of the tumor layer by layer while examining each layer under a microscope. This precise method offers an extremely high cure rate and minimizes damage to healthy tissue.

8. Psoralen Plus Ultraviolet A (PUVA) Therapy: PUVA therapy combines the use of a photosensitizing drug (psoralen) with exposure to UVA light. It is primarily used for conditions like psoriasis, eczema, and vitiligo.

9. Skin Grafts and Flap Surgery: For extensive skin diseases, surgeons may perform grafts or flap surgery. This involves removing damaged skin and replacing it with healthy skin taken from another part of the body (graft) or nearby tissue (flap).

10. Targeted Therapies: Some skin diseases, such as skin cancer, may require targeted therapies that aim to block specific molecules involved in the disease's growth and progression. These therapies are personalized to the patient's specific genetic and molecular makeup.

Professional treatments play a critical role in managing skin diseases. Dermatologists and healthcare providers are equipped to evaluate, diagnose, and recommend the most appropriate treatments based on the individual's condition and needs. These treatments offer hope and relief for those living with skin diseases, and they continue to advance with emerging technologies and research, ultimately improving outcomes for patients.

10.2 INNOVATIVE SKIN CARE TRENDS

The field of dermatology and skin care is constantly evolving, driven by advancements in technology, research, and consumer demand for effective solutions. Innovative skin care trends have emerged in recent years, offering new approaches to managing skin diseases and improving overall skin health.

1. Tele-Dermatology: Tele-dermatology has gained significant momentum, especially in the wake of the COVID-19 pandemic. It allows patients to consult with dermatologists remotely, providing accessible and convenient care. This trend enables early diagnosis and treatment for various skin diseases while reducing the need for in-person visits.

2. Artificial Intelligence (AI) in Skin Disease Diagnosis: AI is transforming dermatology by helping with the early detection of skin diseases. Machine learning algorithms can analyze images of skin lesions and provide quick, accurate assessments. AI-driven applications are becoming valuable tools for both patients and dermatologists.

3. Personalized Skin Care: The concept of personalized skin care is expanding. Tailored treatments based on an individual's skin type, genetics, and specific skin concerns are gaining traction. These customized approaches ensure that skin care regimens are better aligned with a person's unique needs.

4. Microbiome-focused Products: Emerging research has shed light on the importance of the skin microbiome—the community of microorganisms living on the skin's surface. Innovative skin care products now incorporate prebiotics, probiotics, and postbiotics to promote a balanced and healthy skin microbiome, aiding in conditions such as acne and eczema.

5. At-Home Skin Testing Kits: Various companies are offering at-home skin testing kits that allow individuals to analyze their skin's unique characteristics. These tests provide valuable insights into factors like hydration levels, collagen density, and sensitivity, guiding people in choosing the most suitable skin care products.

6. Digital Apps for Skin Monitoring: Mobile apps equipped with AI technology are used to monitor skin conditions and changes over time. Users can track moles for signs of melanoma, evaluate acne severity, or monitor conditions like eczema. These apps encourage proactive skin care management.

7. Eco-friendly and Sustainable Skin Care: As environmental consciousness grows, sustainable and eco-friendly skin care products are becoming more popular. Consumers are seeking skin care items with minimal packaging waste and environmentally friendly sourcing and production.

8. Nanotechnology in Skin Care: Nanotechnology is revolutionizing skin care by allowing for the creation of nano-sized particles that can penetrate the skin more effectively. This innovation enhances the delivery of active ingredients, making skin care products more efficient in addressing skin diseases.

9. Wearable Skin Sensors: Wearable technology has extended into the realm of skin care with sensors that monitor skin health and exposure to harmful environmental factors. These devices can alert individuals to UV radiation levels, pollution, or even skin hydration status.

10. Skin-focused Nutraceuticals:

Nutraceuticals, which are a blend of nutrition and pharmaceuticals, are becoming popular for addressing skin diseases. These supplements contain ingredients like vitamins, antioxidants, and botanical extracts that support skin health from within.

These innovative skin care trends reflect the growing demand for effective, convenient, and personalized solutions in the field of dermatology. As technology and research continue to advance, the future of skin care holds promise for improved skin disease management and overall skin health. Consulting a dermatologist or healthcare professional is essential for navigating these trends and making informed choices regarding skin care and disease management.

CHAPTER 11

<u>SKIN CARE FOR ALL SEASONS</u>

Proper skin care is essential throughout the year to maintain healthy, radiant skin and manage skin diseases effectively. Each season brings its unique challenges and considerations for skin health. By adapting your skin care routine to the changing seasons, you can better address specific concerns and keep skin diseases in check.

Winter:
Winter often comes with cold, dry air that can lead to skin dryness and exacerbate conditions like eczema. To combat this, use richer, heavier moisturizers to lock in moisture.

Additionally, minimize hot showers and use lukewarm water, as hot water can strip the skin's natural oils. Don't forget sunscreen even in winter, as UV rays can still harm the skin.

Spring:

With spring's arrival, focus on skin renewal. Exfoliate to remove dead winter skin cells and promote a fresher complexion. Consider using lighter, hydrating products as the weather warms. Allergies can also trigger skin issues, so manage allergies effectively to prevent skin conditions like hives or dermatitis.

Summer:

Sun protection is paramount in summer. Apply a broad-spectrum sunscreen with at least SPF 30 to guard against UV damage. Light, oil-free, and non-comedogenic products are best to prevent clogged pores. Heat and humidity can exacerbate acne, so maintain a consistent cleansing routine.

Fall:

As the weather cools down, it's essential to transition to a more hydrating skin care routine. Cooler air can be drying, so opt for a thicker moisturizer to combat dryness and flakiness. Don't neglect your lips; use a lip balm with SPF to protect against UV radiation.

Year-round:

Regardless of the season, there are universal practices for managing skin diseases and maintaining skin health. Regularly cleanse your skin with a gentle, pH-balanced cleanser. Apply moisturizer, even in warm weather, as it helps maintain skin hydration. Use fragrance-free products, especially if you have sensitive skin, to minimize irritation.

For skin diseases like eczema, psoriasis, or acne, work closely with a dermatologist who can provide targeted treatments, such as topical medications or therapies. Stay hydrated by drinking enough water, as proper hydration is crucial for overall skin health.

Skin care should be a year-round commitment. Pay attention to your skin's changing needs as the seasons shift, and make adjustments to your routine accordingly. By doing so, you can effectively manage skin diseases and

keep your skin looking its best
throughout the year.

11.1 SEASONAL SKIN CARE ADJUSTMENTS

Seasonal skin care adjustments are crucial for maintaining healthy, vibrant skin year-round. Each season brings unique challenges, and adapting your skincare regimen accordingly can help prevent common issues and ensure your skin remains in optimal condition.

WINTER:

During the winter months, cold and dry air can lead to dry, flaky skin. To combat this, make these adjustments:

1. Hydration: Use a richer, more emollient moisturizer to lock in moisture and provide a protective barrier against the cold wind.

2. Gentle Cleansing: Opt for a mild, hydrating cleanser to avoid stripping the skin of essential oils. Avoid hot showers, as they can further dry out the skin.

3. Sunscreen: Don't forget sunscreen, as UV rays can still harm the skin in winter, especially when reflected off snow.

SPRING:

Spring often brings seasonal allergies and increased pollen, which can exacerbate skin issues:

1. **Exfoliation:** Exfoliate to remove dead skin cells and promote a fresh complexion after the winter season.

2. **Allergy Management:** Manage allergies effectively to prevent skin conditions like hives or dermatitis.

3. **Lighter Products:** Consider using lighter, hydrating products as the weather warms.

SUMMER:

The summer heat and sun require specialized adjustments to your skincare routine:

1. **Sun Protection:** Apply a broad-spectrum sunscreen with at least SPF 30 to shield against UV damage.

2. Oil-Free Products: Use light, oil-free, and non-comedogenic products to prevent clogged pores in the heat and humidity.

3. Acne Prevention: The heat and humidity can exacerbate acne, so maintain a consistent cleansing routine.

FALL:

Cooler weather and dryer air can affect the skin:

1. Hydration: Transition to a thicker moisturizer to combat dryness and flakiness.

2. Lip Care: Don't neglect your lips; use a lip balm with SPF to protect against UV radiation and dryness.

YEAR-ROUND:

Regardless of the season, some skincare practices should remain consistent:

1. Cleansing: Regularly cleanse your skin with a gentle, pH-balanced cleanser.

2. Moisturization: Apply moisturizer daily to help maintain skin hydration.

3. Fragrance-Free: Use fragrance-free products, especially if you have sensitive skin, to minimize irritation.

4. Consult a Dermatologist: If you have skin diseases or persistent concerns, work with a dermatologist who can provide targeted treatments and advice on your skincare regimen.

Adapting your skincare routine to seasonal changes ensures that your skin stays in its best possible condition throughout the year. Understanding your skin's changing needs and making necessary adjustments can help you avoid common issues and maintain healthy, radiant skin.

11.2 PROTECTING YOUR SKIN YEAR-ROUND

Guarding your skin time- round is essential for maintaining its health and beauty while precluding a range of skin issues. The key to effective skin protection lies in a comprehensive approach that considers colorful factors, anyhow of the season. Then is a companion to help you guard your skin throughout the time.

1. Sunscreen Is Your Stylish Friend

Time- round sun protection isnon- negotiable. UV radiation can harm your skin in all seasons, leading to unseasonable aging, skin cancer, and other issues. Apply a broad- diapason sunscreen with at least SPF 30 daily, indeed on cloudy days. Reapply every two hours when outside, and do not forget to cover your lips and cognizance.

2. Stay Doused

Proper hydration is vital for healthy skin. Drinking an acceptable quantum of water keeps your skin moisturized and helps flush out poisons. Strive to drink a minimum of eight glasses of water every day. In the colder months, use a humidifier to combat inner heating that can dry out the air and your skin.

3. Maintain a Healthy Diet

Your skin's appearance is nearly tied to your diet. Consume a variety of fruits, vegetables, spare proteins, and healthy fats. Omega- 3 adipose acids, set up in fish and flaxseeds, are particularly salutary for your skin. Antioxidant-rich foods, like berries and dark leafy flora, help combat free revolutionaries that can damage your skin.

4. Gentle Cleansing

Use a gentle, pH- balanced cleaner for your face and body. Harsh detergents can strip your skin of essential canvases , leading to blankness and vexation. Avoid hot showers, as they can have the same effect.

5. Acceptable Sleep

Sleep is pivotal for skin rejuvenescence and form. Aim for 7- 8 hours of quality sleep each night to maintain your skin's health and radiance.

6. Stress operation

habitual stress can complicate skin issues like acne and psoriasis. Incorporate stress operation ways similar as contemplation, deep breathing exercises, and regular physical exertion into your diurnal routine.

7. Seasonal adaptations

acclimatize your skincare routine to the changing seasons. In downtime, use a richer moisturizer to combat blankness; in summer, prioritize oil painting-free products to help clogged pores. slip in the spring to remove dead skin cells and promote renewal.

8. cover Against Environmental Factors

Environmental adulterants can harm your skin. Use antioxidant-rich skincare products to shield against these adulterants. Wearing defensive apparel and headdresses when necessary can also minimize exposure.

9. Dermatologist Consultation

still, consult a dermatologist, If you have skin conditions or patient enterprises. They can give targeted treatments, similar as topical specifics or advanced curatives, acclimatized to your specific requirements.

10. No Smoking

Smoking accelerates the aging process and contributes to colorful skin issues, including wrinkles and poor crack mending. Quitting smoking can significantly ameliorate your skin's health.

Time-round skin protection requires a harmonious and holistic approach. By following these guidelines and making necessary adaptations throughout the seasons, you can insure your skin remains healthy, vibrant, and resistant to colorful skin conditions and conditions.

www.ingramcontent.com/pod-product-compliance
Lightning Source LLC
Chambersburg PA
CBHW050805260726
48660CB00004B/1265